THE CUTTER INCIDENT

THE CUTTER
INCIDENT

How America's First Polio Vaccine

Led to the Growing Vaccine Crisis

Paul A. Offit, M.D.

Yale University Press   New Haven and London

Set in Stemple Garamond type by Keystone Typesetting, Inc.
Printed in the United States of America by R. R. Donnelley & Sons.

The Library of Congress has cataloged the hardcover edition as follows:
Offit, Paul A.
The Cutter incident : how America's first polio vaccine led to the growing vaccine crisis /
Paul A. Offit.
p. cm.
Includes bibliographical references and index.
ISBN 0-300-10864-8 (cloth : alk. paper)
1. Poliomyelitis vaccine—History. 2. Poliomyelitis—Vaccination—United States—History.
3. Cutter Laboratories. 4. Vaccines—United States. I. Title.
QR189.5.P6044 2005
614.5'49'0973—dc22
2005040105

ISBN 978-0-300-12605-1 (pbk. : alk. paper)

A catalogue record for this book is available from the British Library.

The paper in this book meets the guidelines for permanence and durability of the Committee
on Production Guidelines for Book Longevity of the Council on Library Resources.

For Bonnie
and for our children,
Will and Emily

The mass and majesty of this world, all
  That carries weight and always weighs the same
Lay in the hands of others; they were small
  And could not hope for help, and no help came

W. H. Auden

Contents

Prologue

We live longer than we used to. During the twentieth century, the lifespan of Americans increased by thirty years. Much of the increase was caused by such advances as antibiotics, purified drinking water, sanitation, safer workplaces, better nutrition, safer foods, seatbelts, and a decline in smoking. But no single medical advance had a greater impact on human health than vaccines. Before vaccines, Americans could expect that every year measles would infect 4 million children and kill three thousand; diphtheria would kill fifteen thousand people, mostly teenagers; rubella (German measles) would cause twenty thousand babies to be born blind, deaf, or mentally retarded; pertussis (whooping cough) would kill eight thousand children, most of whom were less than one year old; and polio would permanently paralyze fifteen thousand children and kill one thousand. Because of vaccines most of these diseases have been completely or virtually eliminated from the United States. Smallpox—a disease estimated to have killed 500 million people—was eradicated by vaccines.

Despite their success, vaccines are in trouble; only four companies now make them, and two of the four have severely reduced their vaccine research programs. The result has been an unrelenting series of vaccine shortages and a lack of hope that certain vaccines will ever be made. Recent examples show just how bad things have gotten: In 1998, the tetanus vaccine was in such short supply that its use was restricted to emergency rooms. Since 2000, a vaccine to prevent the most common cause of severe pneumonia, bloodstream infections, and meningitis in children (pneumococcus) has been available only intermittently.

During these shortages, when the vaccine has been difficult or impossible to obtain, parents could only hope that their children weren't among the thousands permanently harmed or killed by pneumococcus every year.

The influenza epidemic in 2003–2004 started earlier than usual and created a demand for influenza vaccine that dramatically exceeded supply. During that epidemic 36,000 people, including 152 children, died from influenza. In 2004–2005 the situation worsened: 30 million fewer doses of influenza vaccine were available to the United States than the year before.

Since 1998, there have been severe shortages of nine of the twelve vaccines routinely given to young children. All these shortages resulted in delays in administering vaccines, and some children never received the vaccines they missed.

Why are pharmaceutical companies abandoning vaccines? Part of the answer is rooted in one largely forgotten incident that occurred fifty years ago, when a small pharmaceutical company in northern California made a vaccine that caused an epidemic affecting thousands of people. It was one of the worst biological disasters in American history, exploded the myth of the invulnerability of science and destroyed faith in the vaccine enterprise. As a consequence, juries handed down verdicts to make sure that it never happened again. Ironically, those legal precedents caused pharmaceutical companies to abandon existing vaccines and to reduce their efforts to develop new ones.

Introduction

I thought her ponytail was pulled too tight.
—Josephine Gottsdanker

ON MONDAY AFTERNOON, APRIL 18, 1955, JOSE-
phine Gottsdanker drove her five-year-old daughter, Anne, and ten-
year-old son, Jerry, to the pediatrician. Several days earlier Josephine,
an intense, bespectacled, highly educated woman, had watched the
television program *See It Now,* in which Edward R. Murrow, a CBS
News correspondent, had interviewed Jonas Salk, the scientist who
had just developed a polio vaccine. Josephine wanted Salk's new vaccine for her children. In the doctor's office she watched the nurse take
a vial of vaccine out of the refrigerator, draw the vaccine into a prop-
erly sterilized glass syringe, and inject it into the muscle of Anne's
upper right leg. Minutes later, the procedure was repeated for her son.

Summer was near, and Josephine Gottsdanker, like most American
mothers in the 1950s, was afraid. She was afraid of other children. And
she was afraid of swimming pools, water fountains, city streets, recre-
ational camps, and neighbors' houses. She was afraid that this summer
her children would be among the tens of thousands claimed every year
by polio.

The tragedies caused by polio were fierce and unrelenting. "It was
an atmosphere of grief, terror, and helpless rage," remembered a nurse
who worked on the medical wards at a Pittsburgh hospital. "It was
horrible. I remember a high school boy weeping because he was completely paralyzed and couldn't move a hand to kill himself. I remember
paralyzed women in iron lungs giving birth to normal babies." A
daughter whose mother was a victim of polio in Phoenix, Arizona,
remembered that during her "first night in the hospital, when the virus

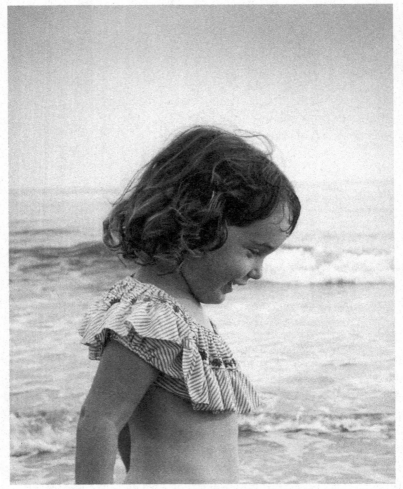

Anne Gottsdanker, September 1953 (courtesy of Anne
Gottsdanker).

had raged through her body, deadening muscle after muscle but leaving her on fire with pain, doctors performed an emergency trache-
otomy to keep her from suffocating. Her throat muscles useless, she
was unable to breathe, cough, or swallow on her own." "It was 1943,"
a former camper remembered. "We were on Schroon lake in New York
State at a camp for boys called Idylwold. Four of the boys got polio
that summer. One day no one could find our head counselor, Bill Lilly.
He took what happened to those boys pretty hard. The police were

called and, after they searched all around the lake, they found that Bill had hung himself from a tree—hung himself. We were all huddled around the beach when the police came to tell us. I'll never forget it."

On April 22, four days after her children were vaccinated, Josephine Gottsdanker loaded her children into the back seat of the car and drove from Santa Barbara, California, to Calexico—a town on the border between California and Mexico—to visit her parents and relatives. The visit was uneventful. But on the afternoon of April 26, during the drive back from Calexico, Josephine noticed that something was wrong with her daughter. "We stopped at a little mountain village for coffee and ice cream, and she said that her head hurt. I thought her ponytail was pulled too tight. It seemed to me like a casual child's complaint at the time. Then she vomited in the car. We took her to County Hospital. By then she had lost motion in the upper part of her leg—then it moved to the lower part."

"I remember my dad taking me out of the car and carrying me to the curb of the hospital," said Anne. "I couldn't move my legs. I was totally paralyzed. I didn't know what was going on, but I was too young to be afraid." Despite receiving Salk's vaccine, Anne Gottsdanker had contracted polio. Jerry, vaccinated from the same vial at the same time as his sister, was fine.

Anne wasn't alone. After receiving Salk's vaccine, forty thousand children developed headaches, neck stiffness, muscle weakness, and fever; about two hundred were permanently and severely paralyzed; and ten died. Most of these children lived in California and Idaho, and most were paralyzed in their arms, even though polio typically paralyzed the legs. Children were getting polio even though polio season was still a few months away. And children given Salk's vaccine were spreading polio to others.

The strange outbreak of polio in the spring of 1955 caused the first national response to a medical emergency, led to the firing of several high-ranking public health officials, pushed federal oversight of vaccines out of its infancy, and resulted in a court case whose verdict eventually threatened the viability of all vaccines. Alexander Langmuir, chief of the Communicable Diseases Center in Atlanta, Georgia, was among the first to realize exactly what was happening. Within days of the outbreak, Langmuir had given the tragedy a name. He called it "the Cutter Incident."

Little White Coffins

There were three little hearses before the door; all her children had been swept away.
—New York City social worker, July 27, 1916

ON JUNE 6, 1916, THE NEW YORK CITY HEALTH DE-partment received reports on two children, John Pamaris and Armanda Schuccjio; both had suddenly developed high fever and paralysis. Two days later, the health department heard about four more children with the same symptoms. All six children were less than eight years old, all lived in Brooklyn, all were born of immigrant Italian parents, and all had polio. By the end of that week, 6 cases had grown to 33; by the end of the following week, 33 had grown to 150. The disease had spread from Brooklyn to all five New York City boroughs.

The man in charge of controlling the outbreak was Haven Emerson. Appointed commissioner of health just one year earlier, Emerson was the son of a physician and the grandnephew of poet Ralph Waldo Emerson. A tall, angular man with thinning hair and a mustache, Emerson was a public health zealot. He was confident that his rigorous control measures would stop the spread of polio. Although sporadic cases of polio had occurred since the fifteenth century B.C., Emerson knew that large outbreaks had never occurred in the United States. In the late 1800s and early 1900s, small outbreaks had occurred in Otter Creek, Vermont; Philadelphia, Pennsylvania; West Feliciana, Louisiana; and Boston, Massachusetts. But America's experience with polio didn't prepare Emerson for what was about to happen in New York City that summer.

Emerson's strategy was two-pronged: promote better sanitation and quarantine suspected cases. He reasoned that polio was a contagious disease and that quarantining people would decrease the spread

4

of infection. (Quarantine, derived from the Italian *quarantina*, meaning "forty," originally referred to the forty days that ships were held at port before passengers—who were feared to carry the plague—could disembark.) Emerson also reasoned that polio, like other infectious diseases, would spread more easily in communities with inadequate plumbing and poor sewage. He described his plan: "All premises housing a case of polio [were to be] placarded and the family quarantined; the windows were to be screened, the bed linen disinfected, nurses were to change their clothing immediately after tending any patient, and household pets were not allowed in any patient's room." Emerson quarantined thousands of children, but many parents imposed their own form of isolation. A social worker recalled, "In one house the window was not only shut, but the cracks were stuffed with rags so that the disease could not come in. The babies had no clothes on, and were so wet and hot that they looked as if they had been dipped in oil, and the flies were sticking all over them."

Few tenement dwellers met the requirements for home quarantine—a private toilet, separate dining facilities, and a private nurse. As a result, children from poorer families were taken to hospitals, often against their parents' will. On August 25, 1916, a story appeared in the *New York Journal:*

> Mrs. Jennie Dasnoit of 365 64th St., Brooklyn, is under the care of a physician today as a result of a strange experience with the infantile paralysis quarantine. Three policemen forced their way into her home, broke down the door to the bedroom, and drew their revolvers in assisting the ambulance surgeon to obtain possession of her small nephew, a paralysis suspect. The child, Cornelius Wilson, two-year-old son of Mrs. Dasnoit's dead sister, is in the Kingston Avenue Hospital, Brooklyn, where the physicians have not yet decided that he is suffering from paralysis.
>
> The policemen entered the house, Mrs. Dasnoit says, by cutting the screen covering a window on the first floor, breaking their way into the room where Mrs. Dasnoit stood with the baby in her arms. Their revolvers were drawn, she charges.
>
> Mrs. Dasnoit's screams attracted neighbors to the house but before they could enter two of the policemen held her while the third pulled the child from her arms and passed him through the window to the surgeon.

Parents fought back. Anna Henry, a nurse employed by the clinic at Public School 91 in Flatbush (Brooklyn), reported to police that she

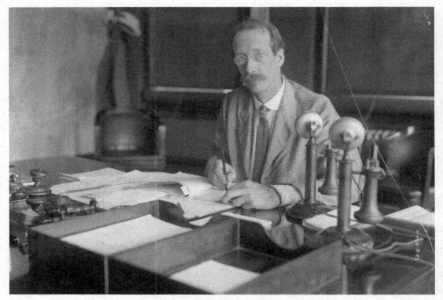

Haven Emerson, New York City health commissioner, July 1916 (courtesy of the Bettmann Archives).

received a letter written in blood: "If you report any more of our babies to the Board of Health we will kill you and nobody will know what happened to you. Keep off our street and don't report our homes and we will do you no harm." At the bottom of the letter, beneath a crude drawing of a skull and crossbones, was the statement: "We will kill you like a dog." Anna Henry was later escorted by the police to and from work.

Haven Emerson believed that the epidemic started because "90 immigrant Italians under the age of ten had [moved to] Brooklyn where the outbreak appeared" and that immigrants were the first to get polio because they were poorer and dirtier. He wanted residents to bathe their children and fix their toilets, yards, cellars, and plumbing. He wanted the city to provide fresh water, collect garbage more frequently, and protect people from flies. Every day janitors and homeowners, under penalty of fine or imprisonment, complied with Emerson's sanitary code; every day 4 million gallons of water washed the streets; every day city workers killed 300–450 cats and dogs because they believed them to harbor germ-carrying fleas; and every day chil-

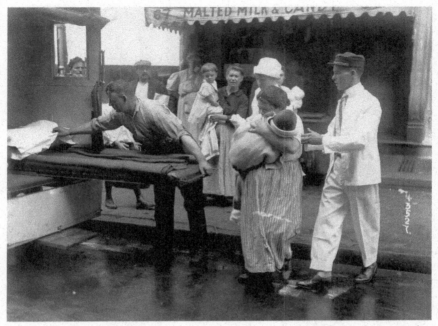

Mother holds child while health attendants prepare ambulance; New York City, 1916. Young polio victims from poorer families were taken to hospitals, often against their parents' will (courtesy of the Bettmann Archives).

dren continued to be paralyzed. During the week of June 24, 1916, polio claimed another 233 children.

On June 30 Emerson said, "We believe that application of well-organized sanitary measures will limit this outbreak." As July 4 approached, he urged parents to keep their children away from others. On July 5 all movie theaters banned children under the age of sixteen. Three days later, carnivals, parades, public picnics, and excursions ceased, leaving the streets deserted. In the following week there were another 700 cases and 170 deaths from polio. The epidemic continued unchecked.

On July 8 an editorial in the *New York Medical Journal* stated, "The plague seems to have reached its height and to be already abating." But the disease wasn't abating. In the week of August 5 there were another 1,200 cases and 370 deaths. Dr. Robert Guilfoy had announced in July that one child died from polio every two and

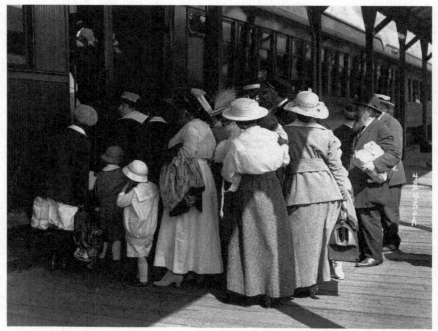

Residents leave New York City, 1916 (courtesy of the Bettmann Archives).

one-half hours; by early August it was every twenty-six minutes. By mid-August, polio had paralyzed 5,500 people and killed 1,500.

Federal authorities, desperate to contain the epidemic, issued a regulation that no child could leave New York City without a certificate for interstate travel. Residents living outside the city panicked. A self-appointed citizens' committee of five hundred in Huntington, Long Island, entered every home in town looking for suspected cases of polio. Residents of Glen Cove, Long Island, threatened to kill the health officer and burn down the hospital after the arrival of several polio patients. Policemen in Hoboken, New Jersey, guarded every entrance to the city with instructions that no one could seek safe haven. At gunpoint, two policemen forced a family of seven to turn back; the family had given up their home in Brooklyn to move to Hoboken.

Isolated and desperate for a cure, New York City residents tried everything. They ingested catnip, skullcap, lady's slipper, earthworm oil, blackberry brandy, and the blood of frogs, snakes, and horses. Following a rumor about the wondrous powers of ox blood, parents showed up at East Side slaughterhouses with buckets. They hung charms around their necks made of pepper, garlic, camphor, and onions. A former state legislator sold cedar wood shavings to be worn around the neck "to protect the child from death and . . . prevent germs [and] insects from attacking the victim," and one man sold "Sol," containing sassafras and alcohol, to "cure infantile paralysis." Both men spent thirty days in jail for making false claims.

Doctors, similarly desperate, injected adrenaline or fresh human saliva into the spinal fluid or took spinal fluid from infected people and injected it back under the skin. One physician, George Retan, claimed dramatic success with a technique that involved inserting a large hollow needle into a child's back, draining spinal fluid, and at the same time infusing large quantities of salt solution into a vein. Retan reasoned that his technique washed poisons out of the nervous system. With wider use—when the treatment killed more people than it saved—physicians abandoned the procedure.

During the last three weeks of August, polio paralyzed 3,500 people and killed 900. Typically, polio killed 5 percent of its victims, but in New York City in the summer of 1916, for reasons that remain unclear, 27 percent of those infected died.

Two years after the New York City polio epidemic, influenza killed 675,000 Americans—more than the combined number of American deaths in World War I, World War II, and the Vietnam War. Although the influenza deaths far outnumbered the polio deaths, polio was in many ways more devastating. People infected with influenza either died from pneumonia or recovered, but children paralyzed by polio rarely recovered. The sight of small children trying to use withered arms or struggling to walk with crutches or lying helplessly in breathing machines (called iron lungs) was a constant, crushing reminder of the infection.

By late September 1916 the number of new cases of polio finally declined, and New York City schools reopened. When the epidemic was over, polio had paralyzed more than 9,000 people and killed 2,400; most were children less than ten years old. It was the largest epidemic of polio ever recorded. One year later, the New York City Health Department reported that the world's knowledge of polio "was based

on a smaller number of autopsies recorded in the whole medical litera-
ture than were performed at one of the department's hospitals during
the past summer."

Months later, Haven Emerson admitted defeat: "There is no positive proof that a demonstrable amount of protection or prevention
resulted from the general measures enforced." Emerson had assumed
incorrectly that by quarantining infected children and promoting better sanitation he could stop the spread of polio. But polio was different
from other infections.

New York City residents didn't know what caused polio. They blamed
fish, milk, fleas, rats, cats, horses, mosquitoes, chickens, shark vapors,
pasteurized milk, wireless electricity, radio waves, tobacco smoke, au-
tomobile exhaust, doctors' beards, organ grinders' monkeys, and poi-
sonous gases from Europe. They blamed parents for tickling their
children. They blamed tarantulas for injecting poisons into bananas.
Although unknown to most New York City residents, the cause of
polio had already been discovered.

On November 18, 1908, eight years before the polio epidemic in
New York City, Karl Landsteiner, a doctor in Vienna, Austria, found
the cause of polio. An intense, solitary man who kept a death mask of
his mother on the wall above his bed, Landsteiner performed an au-
topsy on a nine-year-old Viennese boy who had died of polio. He
removed the boy's spinal cord, ground it up, and injected it into two
monkeys; soon both monkeys were paralyzed. When Landsteiner removed the spinal cords from the monkeys, sliced them into thin sec-
tions, and looked at them under a microscope, he found that they
looked just like the spinal cords from children who had been killed by
polio. Landsteiner reasoned that polio was caused by a virus that was
present in the boy's spinal cord.

Three years after Landsteiner's discovery, Carl Kling, a twenty-
four-year-old Swede working at the State Bacteriological Institute,
figured out how polio virus was spread. During an outbreak in Sweden
that paralyzed four thousand people, Kling examined the hearts, lungs,
spinal cords, throats, and intestines of fourteen children who had
died of polio. He duplicated Landsteiner's findings by showing that
ground-up spinal cords from these children paralyzed monkeys. That

wasn't a surprising discovery, but Kling also found that fluids taken from the throats, windpipes, and intestines of these children also paralyzed monkeys. He reasoned that polio might be spread from one person to another by a virus present in the saliva or intestines of people who were infected. At the time Kling performed his studies, polio had a range of symptoms that included sore throat and fever (mild polio); stiff neck, mild paralysis, and headache (abortive polio); permanent paralysis of the arms and legs (paralytic polio); and paralysis of the muscles necessary for breathing (bulbar polio). But Kling also found that in some instances polio was present in the throats and intestines of people *who didn't have any symptoms* (asymptomatic polio). Kling's observations explained why Haven Emerson couldn't stop the spread of polio in New York City by quarantining only people who were paralyzed by the disease: most people who were spreading polio weren't sick.

The next important discovery—and one that offered a ray of hope that polio could be prevented—was made by Simon Flexner, director of the Rockefeller Institute for Medical Research in New York City. Working at the same time as Carl Kling, Flexner took blood from monkeys who were recovering from polio and let it clot; the fraction of blood not contained in the clot was called serum. He then inoculated monkeys with a mixture of serum and polio-infected spinal cords. Typically monkeys inoculated with polio-infected spinal cords got polio. But to Flexner's surprise, with the addition of serum to the spinal cords before inoculation, polio virus didn't paralyze the monkeys. He called what he found in the serum from previously infected animals "germicidal substances." Today we call these "substances" antibodies.

Thirty years after Flexner had identified polio antibodies, a team of researchers at Johns Hopkins Hospital in Baltimore revealed more of polio's secrets. They determined that polio virus entered the body through the mouth and traveled to the intestines and then to the blood. They found, as had Carl Kling, that most people with polio virus in their intestines and blood never developed symptoms of polio. But in some people (and this could be as rare as 1 in 150 infected people), polio virus traveled from the blood to the spinal cord, entered the cells of the spinal cord, and made more polio virus particles. (A cell is the smallest structural unit that is capable of independent function.

Organs such as the liver, spleen, brain, and spinal cord are composed of billions of cells.) In the process of reproducing itself in the cells of the spinal cord, polio virus destroyed the spinal cord and caused paralysis. The Hopkins researchers showed that polio virus had to enter the blood to get to the spinal cord. Thus if researchers could find a way to induce polio antibodies in blood, the antibodies could neutralize polio virus *before* it got to the spinal cord.

To understand what polio was and how it was spread, Landsteiner, Kling, Flexner, and the Hopkins researchers relied on monkeys. Working with monkeys was expensive, dangerous, and slow. But monkeys paved the way to the first ill-fated polio vaccines.

By the early 1900s it was apparent that people who were infected with polio were usually immune to a second infection. The task for polio researchers was clear: find a way to induce immunity without causing disease. The first researchers who tried to make a polio vaccine were John Kolmer of Philadelphia and Maurice Brodie of New York. Between 1934 and 1935, Kolmer and Brodie inoculated seventeen thousand children with their vaccines. At the time that Kolmer and Brodie made their vaccines, three viral vaccines had already been made. Each used a different strategy, but all used the same concept: separate a virus's capacity to cause disease from its capacity to induce antibodies that protected against disease.

The first vaccine, developed by Edward Jenner, a country doctor in southwest England in the late 1700s, was made to prevent the world's most contagious and fatal disease: smallpox. In Jenner's time, smallpox killed more people than all other infectious diseases combined. During the eighteenth century, it killed four hundred thousand people worldwide every year; the virus caused blindness in 30 percent of those who survived and disfigurement in almost all.

Jenner was the sixth son of Stephan Jenner, the vicar of Berkeley. After training with the noted surgeon John Hunter, Jenner rejected lucrative offers to remain in London and returned to work among the farmers and local tradesmen near his home in Bristol. In 1770, during a local outbreak of smallpox, a dairymaid came to Dr. Jenner and said that she wouldn't get sick because she already had had "cowpox," a disease of cows that caused blisters on their udders. People who milked cows infected with cowpox often developed these same blisters on their hands. The dairymaid reasoned that cowpox protected her from smallpox—a belief shared by many local farmers.

On May 14, 1796, in a small hut outside of Bristol, Edward Jenner tested the milkmaid's theory. He inoculated a young boy with pus from a cowpox blister taken from the hand of a milkmaid. Later, to see if the procedure had worked, Jenner inoculated the boy with crusts from the blister of someone infected with smallpox. The little boy survived.

In June 1798, delighted with his findings, Jenner wrote a paper entitled "An Inquiry into the Causes and Effects of the Variolae Vaccinae, a Disease Discovered in Some of the Western Counties of England Particularly Glouchestershire, and Known by the Name of 'Cowpox.'" The term "Variolae Vaccinae," literally "smallpox of the cow," was later shortened to "vaccination." Immediately recognized for their significance, Jenner's observations were translated into six languages, and his technique of vaccination was used throughout the world. By 1977, smallpox, a disease that had killed hundreds of millions of people, was eliminated from the face of the earth.

The world's second vaccine, made by Louis Pasteur, prevented rabies, a disease transmitted by the bite of an infected (rabid) animal. People feared rabies because its symptoms were unrelenting and death was inevitable. Like polio virus, rabies virus infected the spinal cord. Thus Pasteur took spinal cords from people who had been killed by rabies, ground them up, and injected them into rabbits. All of the rabbits developed rabies and died. However, when Pasteur first dried out the infected spinal cords, the rabbits didn't die. Rabies virus appeared to be susceptible to drying.

Pasteur got a chance to test his vaccine on July 6, 1885. Several days earlier, a rabid dog had savagely bitten a nine-year-old boy, Joseph Meister, and Meister's mother begged Pasteur to save her son. Pasteur inoculated the boy with a preparation of infected rabbit spinal cord that had been dried for fifteen days (a process that rendered the virus incapable of causing disease in rabbits). During the next ten days, Meister was given twelve successive inoculations with rabbit spinal cords that had each been less dried out (and were therefore more dangerous) than those used for the previous inoculations. Meister survived. Working as a gatekeeper for the Pasteur Institute in Paris, he lived until 1940.

One hundred and twenty years after Jenner developed a smallpox vaccine and forty years after Pasteur developed a rabies vaccine, Max Theiler and Hugo Smith made the world's third vaccine. It protected against yellow fever, a disease that damaged the liver and caused jaundice, a yellowing of the skin. The yellow fever virus also attacked the heart and kidneys and killed about half of those who were infected. Because the virus caused severe internal bleeding (hemorrhaging), it was called a viral hemorrhagic fever. In the 1700s and 1800s, yellow fever commonly led to death in the United States. An outbreak in Philadelphia in the late 1700s killed 10 percent of the city's residents, and an outbreak in New Orleans in the mid-1800s killed 30 percent. The terror it caused can be seen today in response to another viral hemorrhagic fever—Ebola virus.

In the mid-1930s Max Theiler and Hugo Smith, working at the Rockefeller Institute in New York City, made a yellow fever vaccine by serially growing the virus in eggs. After the virus had been passed two hundred times from one egg to the next, they found that it no longer caused disease. Theiler and Smith had successfully weakened yellow fever virus. In the late 1930s Theiler and Smith inoculated more than five hundred thousand Brazilians with their vaccine, and epidemics of yellow fever in Brazil abated. For his work on yellow fever vaccine, Max Theiler won the Nobel Prize in Medicine in 1951 (and always regretted that Hugo Smith was not named as a co-recipient).

Three different strategies had been used successfully to make three different viral vaccines. To make their polio vaccines, Kolmer and Brodie had the option (like Jenner) of taking a nonhuman virus (cowpox) to protect against a related human virus (smallpox), but polio virus caused disease only in humans. They could use Pasteur's idea of drying the virus, but polio virus wasn't susceptible to drying. Or they could use Theiler and Smith's idea of weakening the virus by serially growing it in eggs, but polio virus didn't grow in eggs. So they each tried something else.

John Kolmer was "a quiet, unassuming, earnest little man" who graduated from the University of Pennsylvania School of Medicine in 1908.

Physicians knew Kolmer as the man who had developed the blood test for syphilis (called the Kolmer test). But the press and public knew Kolmer as the doctor who tried to save the life of Calvin Coolidge's son, Calvin Jr.

On the afternoon of June 30, 1924, sixteen-year-old Calvin Coolidge Jr. played several sets of tennis with his brother, John, and two White House doctors. Because he had chosen to wear tennis shoes without socks, Cal Jr. soon developed a blister on his right foot. The blister became infected with a bacterium called *Staphylococcus,* and after a few days Cal Jr. had a high fever, chills, and difficulty breathing; delirious, he begged his father to save his life. Coolidge responded by calling one of the country's leading microbiologists, John Kolmer. Kolmer treated Cal Jr. by injecting him with an antitoxin against *Staphylococcus*—a preparation made by injecting horses with the bacteria, removing their blood, and collecting the serum. But the antitoxin didn't work. Coolidge later recalled: "When he went, the power and glory of the presidency went with him. I do not know why such a price was exacted for occupying the White House."

In 1932, after a severe polio epidemic in Philadelphia, John Kolmer turned his attention to making a polio vaccine. He felt his best chance was to find a chemical that would weaken but not kill the virus. After trying many different agents, he settled on ricinoleate, a substance found in the oil of the castor bean plant (castor oil). To prepare his vaccine, Kolmer took spinal cords from monkeys infected with polio, ground them up, suspended them in a salt solution, filtered them through a fine mesh, and treated them with ricinoleate for fifteen days. After injecting the vaccine into his eleven-year-old son; his fifteen-year-old son; his assistant, Anna Rule; and twenty-five children "convalescing from various medical and surgical ailments," John Kolmer declared his vaccine to be safe.

In the fall of 1934, Kolmer began injecting more than ten thousand children with his vaccine. Given that the spinal cord from one monkey made about forty doses, the size of this study—and the number of monkeys that died in its name—was remarkable.

Unlike Kolmer, Maurice Brodie was just starting a career in medicine and science. Full of energy, "optimistic, and hard-working," Brodie made his vaccine by treating spinal cords from paralyzed monkeys

with formaldehyde for twelve days. Brodie reasoned that formaldehyde, unlike Kolmer's ricinoleate, would kill polio virus and that
killed virus would induce polio antibodies. In the summer of 1934,
after taking a job at New York University and the New York City
Health Department, Brodie inoculated himself and five coworkers.
"As it was now evident that the vaccine could be given with perfect
safety," Brodie proceeded to inoculate twelve children and found that
they developed polio antibodies without developing polio. Brodie was
confident that his vaccine worked and that it was safe. During the next
year, he inoculated seven thousand children with his formaldehyde-
treated polio vaccine.

On a brisk morning in November 1935 in St. Louis, Missouri,
hundreds of physicians, scientists, and public health officials packed
into a meeting of the American Public Health Association to hear John
Kolmer and Maurice Brodie report their results. Chief among those in
attendance was Thomas Rivers, head of the laboratory for the study of
viral diseases at the Rockefeller Institute. "A short, blunt-spoken, self-
professed country boy from Georgia," Rivers had single-handedly
established the study of viruses as a separate field, and by 1935 the
Rockefeller Institute was the center for viral research in the United
States. Almost everyone who trained in the field of virology trained in
Thomas Rivers's laboratory.

Kolmer spoke first. He said that since April 1935 three doses of his
vaccine had been given to ten thousand children in thirty-six states and
Canada. Unfortunately, Kolmer didn't have a control group (children
who had not been inoculated with vaccine) for comparison, so it was
almost impossible to tell whether his vaccine was working. Worse,
several children developed polio soon after getting Kolmer's vaccine.
Sally Gittenberg, a five-year-old from Newark, New Jersey, was injected with a dose of Kolmer's vaccine in her left arm on July 3. On
July 15, she developed fever, headaches, a stiff neck, and vomiting.
Four days later, her left arm was completely paralyzed. Hugh McDon-
nell, a five-year-old from Plainfield, New Jersey, was injected with a
dose of Kolmer's vaccine in his left arm on August 1. On September 7,
he developed paralysis of his left arm and died two days later. Esther
Pfaff, a twenty-one-month-old from Westfield, New Jersey, was injected with a dose of Kolmer's vaccine in the right arm on August 24.

On the night of September 11, Esther couldn't move her right arm. Four days later she was dead. David Costuma, an eight-year-old from Plainfield, New Jersey, was injected with a dose of Kolmer's vaccine in his right arm on August 24. On September 4, with headaches, tremors, and complete paralysis of his right arm, David was taken to the hospital; the next day, he was dead.

In the end, Kolmer's vaccine paralyzed ten children and killed five. Most children were paralyzed within a few weeks of receiving their first dose, and most were paralyzed in the arm that was inoculated. At the St. Louis meeting, Henry Vaughn, the commissioner of health for Detroit, confronted Kolmer with the facts that the vaccinated child in Newark was the only case of polio reported in July and that the two children vaccinated in Plainfield were the only two cases to die from polio in the city. Kolmer countered that the cases were caused by natural polio, not his vaccine. "I do not personally believe that the vaccine was responsible for these cases," he said.

Angered by Kolmer's denials, James Leake, medical director of the Public Health Service in Washington, D.C., rose to speak. Leake was a quick-tempered veteran of the polio wars whose field service dated back to the epidemic in New York City in 1916. Thomas Rivers recalled what happened next: "Jimmy Leake then point-blank accused Kolmer of being a murderer. [He] used the strongest language that I have ever heard at a scientific meeting and when he got through speaking, both vaccines were dead. When you say someone is committing murder people usually stop and think." Kolmer was humiliated: "Gentlemen, this is one time I wish the floor would open up and swallow me."

Maurice Brodie's polio vaccine trial included vaccinated and unvaccinated children (controls) in North Carolina, Virginia, and California. The inclusion of a control group allowed Brodie to figure out whether his vaccine was working. He reported that 5 of 4,500 children who didn't receive his vaccine contracted polio, but only 1 of 7,000 children who did receive it became ill with the disease. This meant that the vaccine was 88 percent effective in preventing polio. But Brodie's description of one case was worrisome: a twenty-year-old vaccinated man developed paralysis in the inoculated arm and died four days later. Several months after the St. Louis meeting, a report by James Leake in a medical journal further questioned whether Brodie's vaccine worked and whether it was safe. Two children, five and fifteen months old, developed polio within two weeks of receiving inoculations.

The men involved in the first polio vaccines met dramatically different fates. John Kolmer continued to publish many papers in laboratory science, became professor of medicine at Temple University School of Medicine, and retired in 1957. In contrast, Maurice Brodie was fired from his jobs at New York University and the New York City Department of Health. His voice was never heard among polio researchers again. During his days as a young researcher in Montreal, Brodie had received many offers from universities and pharmaceutical companies, but after 1935, he couldn't find a place to work. Eventually he accepted a minor position at Providence Hospital in Detroit. In May 1939, at the age of thirty-six, Maurice Brodie died. Many at the time and since have speculated that he killed himself.

Although unappreciated, Maurice Brodie advanced the field of polio research. He was one of the first to show that formaldehyde could kill polio virus; he was the first to figure out that formaldehyde-treated virus induced polio antibodies in children; he was the first to advance the notion that overtreatment with formaldehyde rendered the virus incapable of inducing polio antibodies; and he was the first to claim that a killed polio virus vaccine might induce long-lived protection. All of these ideas were later championed by a man who, although he never met Maurice Brodie, was a medical student at New York University at the time that Brodie performed his experiments—Jonas Salk.

The vaccine trials of John Kolmer and Maurice Brodie had a chilling effect on polio vaccine research. Twenty years passed before anyone dared to try again.

2

Back to the Drawing Board

Churchill once said that to encounter Franklin Roosevelt, with all his buoyant sparkle, his iridescent personality, and his inner élan, was like opening your first bottle of champagne.
—Doris Kearns Goodwin, *No Ordinary Time*

THE 1916 EPIDEMIC IN NEW YORK CITY HAD MADE polio an American disease. Five years later an event that took place off the coast of New Brunswick, Canada, reinforced that notion.

Franklin Delano Roosevelt, then thirty-nine years old, was visiting his family's summer home on Campobello Island. FDR had been a nominee for vice president, secretary of the navy, and a New York legislator. Flamboyant and charismatic, he "loved to swim and to sail, play tennis, golf; to run in the woods and ride horseback in the fields." Late in the afternoon on August 10, 1921, Roosevelt was sitting at his desk writing letters when he felt a chill. Hoping to avoid a bad cold, he went to bed early. But the following morning the muscles of his right knee were weak; by afternoon he couldn't put any weight on his right leg; by evening he was unable to stand or walk. Doctors were called in, the diagnosis of polio was made, and FDR was paralyzed below the waist for the rest of his life.

FDR was certain that he would recover. Every night, disdaining a crutch or a helping hand, he slowly put one foot in front of the other, drenched in sweat, trying desperately, gamely, unsuccessfully to walk. He experimented with salt-water baths and ultraviolet light, electric currents and positive thinking, complete rest and vigorous massage. Nothing worked. Despite numerous failures, in the fall of 1924 FDR was convinced that he had found his cure. Intrigued by the story of Louis Joseph, FDR visited a resort in Georgia called Warm Springs. Joseph, a polio victim, claimed that after swimming in Warm Springs for three summers, he was able to discard his crutches and walk without support. FDR believed that this would happen to him. Within a year, hoping to make it the world's greatest center for the treatment of polio, he bought Warm Springs for $200,000. But FDR never achieved the cure that he sought, and with his ascension to governor of New York and president of the United States, he became increasingly burdened by the ownership of Warm Springs. So he turned to his law partner, Basil O'Connor, for help.

The person most responsible for developing a polio vaccine wasn't Jonas Salk. Nor was it Karl Landsteiner or Simon Flexner or Carl Kling or any of the many researchers, public health officials, or epidemiologists who dedicated their careers to the study and prevention of polio. The person most responsible for eliminating polio from the United States—and later from most of the world—was a Wall Street lawyer named Basil O'Connor.

Daniel Basil ("Doc") O'Connor was a "skinny, frostbitten newsboy [from] the streets of Taunton, Massachusetts" who, after working his way through Dartmouth College and Harvard Law School, became a very successful, very wealthy corporate lawyer. In 1924 O'Connor, recognizing the value of Roosevelt's political connections and influence, convinced him to become his law partner. Three years later, when Roosevelt asked O'Connor to run Warm Springs, he responded by converting it into the Georgia Warm Springs Foundation, a nonprofit organization supported entirely by grants and gifts. The foundation spent all of its money caring for visiting polio victims.

Despite FDR's enormous popularity, the Georgia Warm Springs Foundation struggled. One event saved it. On January 30, 1934, one year after FDR became the thirty-second president of the United States, six thousand balls were held in more than four thousand cities across the United States to celebrate his birthday. Under the slogan "to dance so that others may walk," the events raised more than $1 million. FDR broadcast his thanks during a national radio address: "It is with a humble and thankful heart that I accept this tribute through me to the stricken ones of our great national family. I thank you but lack the words to tell you how deeply I appreciate what you have done and I bid you good night on what is to me the happiest birthday I have ever known." During the next two years, the birthday balls raised an additional $1.3 million. The president's Birthday Ball Commission was born, and for the first time money was spent on polio research.

Now that money was available for research, the Birthday Ball Commission had to find a research director. Their choice was Paul de Kruif. De Kruif had studied bacteriology at the University of Michigan with one of the greatest bacteriologists in the world at the turn of the century, Frederick Novy. After receiving his doctorate, de Kruif moved to New York City to work at the Rockefeller Institute, where he studied the bacteria salmonella, a cause of severe intestinal infection. On the verge of understanding one of the most important phenomena in bacteriology—why some bacteria cause disease and others don't—de Kruif wrote an article for the popular magazine *The Century*. The article, "Our Medicine Men," written anonymously, described physicians as intellectually "flabby," lacking "mental rigor," and never accountable for their mistakes. After learning of the publication, Simon Flexner, the director of the Rockefeller Institute and the man who had first detected polio antibodies, called Paul de Kruif into his office and fired him. As he was leaving the institute, de Kruif commented to a friend that using his "waspish pen," he would get Flexner.

Two years later de Kruif exacted his revenge. He agreed to serve as a consultant to Sinclair Lewis on the book *Arrowsmith*. Set in the fictional McGurk Institute, this was the story of Martin Arrowsmith, a scientist who discovered that certain harmless viruses killed bacteria. (*Arrowsmith* was written ten years before the discovery of antibiotics.) Delighted by his findings, Martin Arrowsmith informed the director of the institute, Dr. A. DeWitt Tubbs, who later stole the credit for Arrowsmith's discovery. De Kruif made sure that all representations in the book were thinly veiled: the McGurk Institute was the Rockefeller Institute; A. DeWitt Tubbs was Simon Flexner; and Martin Arrowsmith was Paul de Kruif. McGurk was a place "in which good scientists might spend an eternity in happy and thoroughly impractical research." Tubbs was "tremendously whiskered on all visible spots save his nose and temples and the palms of his hands, like a Scotch terrier." And Martin Arrowsmith was the earnest, likable hero. Published in 1925, *Arrowsmith* won the Pulitzer Prize and was the most widely read of all of Sinclair Lewis's novels.

One year after the publication of *Arrowsmith*, de Kruif wrote *Microbe Hunters*, a collection of dramatic stories behind the invention of the first microscope, the development of the rabies vaccine, and the discovery of yellow fever virus (among others). *Microbe Hunters* was enormously popular, inspired a generation of young scientists, and launched the career of de Kruif as a writer and journalist. He never worked in a laboratory again.

After the first birthday ball, de Kruif commented to Arthur Carpenter, the manager of the Georgia Warm Springs Foundation, that President Roosevelt was wasting money on it. "Why do you use all that dough to dip cripples in warm water?" asked de Kruif. "That doesn't cure them any more than it cured you or the President. Why don't you ask the President to devote a part of that big dough to research on polio prevention? Nobody knows a thing about that." De Kruif's comments came to the attention of FDR, and in 1934 FDR asked de Kruif to be the chief scientific adviser to the Birthday Ball Commission.

De Kruif was ill suited to direct a research effort. He had been away from research for twelve years. He was not trained as a virologist or an immunologist and knew nothing about polio virus. He was not a physician, had evident disdain for the profession, and knew little about how to perform and evaluate clinical studies. And he was impatient, egotistical, and hot tempered. De Kruif's greatest strength—his ability to popularize science—hardly qualified him to run a scientific organization. His first act as scientific adviser was to fund studies to determine whether spraying acid into children's noses prevented polio virus from entering the body; he hailed nasal spray therapy as "the greatest advance in the fight against infantile paralysis since it was found that the disease could be given to monkeys." In the summer of 1934, doctors sprayed acid into the noses of 4,600 children in Alabama, and in 1937, into the noses of 5,200 children in Toronto. The acid spray didn't prevent children from getting polio, and many permanently lost their sense of smell as a result of the treatment. Later, after failing to show that hormone therapy or vitamins prevented polio, Paul de Kruif quit in a dispute over funds for a nutritionist.

In the fall of 1937, with money running low and preventive strategies proving ineffective or harmful, FDR announced a new foundation to determine "the cause of infantile paralysis and the methods by which it may be prevented." The National Foundation for Infantile Paralysis opened its doors in January 1938.

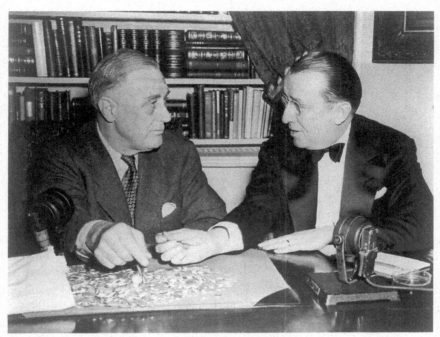

Franklin Delano Roosevelt and Basil O'Connor counting dimes at the
White House (courtesy of the March of Dimes Birth Defects Foundation).

FDR immediately asked Basil O'Connor to be the president of the
National Foundation and to revitalize a research program scarred by
the unsuccessful efforts of Paul de Kruif. O'Connor made the National Foundation one of the most successful public health agencies in
the world. He recruited movie, television, and radio stars to help raise
money; one of them, Eddie Cantor, a vaudevillian known for his bulg-
ing eyes and black-faced minstrel songs, proposed that radio stations
donate thirty seconds of broadcast time for an appeal for money. Cantor planned to ask each of his listeners to donate one dime to the White
House and called the fund-raising campaign "the March of Dimes"—
inspired by a popular newsreel shown in movie theaters, "The March
of Time." After only three days of Cantor's radio appeals, 2,680,000
dimes in more than 200,000 letters arrived at the White House. Within
the year, the foundation raised $1.8 million, mostly in dimes. (This
inspired fund-raising campaign explains why FDR's profile was en-
graved on the face of the dime.)

In addition to direct appeals by celebrities such as Greer Garson, Helen Hayes, Zsa Zsa Gabor, James Cagney, Jack Benny, Kate Smith, Jascha Heifetz, Humphrey Bogart, Willie Mayes, Lucille Ball, Danny Kaye, Bing Crosby, and Mickey Mouse, the National Foundation revolutionized fund-raising by introducing the concept of the "poster child" and making short dramatic films urging people to contribute. One film, *The Crippler,* showed a sinister, shadowy figure spreading over cities and farms, laughing at its victims; it starred the young actress Nancy Davis (later Nancy Reagan). At the end of the movie, ushers carried collection baskets up and down the aisles.

In the early part of the twentieth century, several organizations were dedicated to preventing, treating, and eliminating specific diseases: the National Tuberculosis Association (founded in 1904); the National Society for Crippled Children (now the Easter Seal Society, founded in 1919); and the American Heart Association (founded in 1924). But none were better funded, better staffed, more passionate, or more successful than the National Foundation for Infantile Paralysis (the March of Dimes). At its peak it had three thousand local chapters staffed by ninety thousand year-round volunteers. Between 1938 and 1962 the March of Dimes raised $630 million. Of that sum, $70 million was set aside for research; the rest supported the hospitalization and rehabilitation of every polio victim in America. The money spent by the March of Dimes to understand one disease—ten times more than that spent on polio research by the National Institutes of Health—was unprecedented.

The National Foundation understood that before there could be another vaccine, there was much to learn about polio. With de Kruif gone, O'Connor asked Thomas Rivers, the influential virologist from the Rockefeller Institute, to head the research effort. Rivers compiled a list of eleven research priorities. "Production of a good vaccine" was the last item on the list. Rivers, like many scientists in the late 1930s, was chastened by the failures of John Kolmer and Maurice Brodie; he had given up on a polio vaccine.

At the time that Rivers constructed his list of polio research priorities, two Australians, Macfarlane Burnet and Jane Macnamara, found something that worried polio researchers. Burnet and Macnamara took monkeys and injected them with the MV strain of polio virus, the same strain used by Kolmer and Brodie to make their vaccines. (Polio viruses isolated from different people were referred to as different strains.) After the monkeys recovered from the infection, Burnet and Macnamara again injected them with the MV strain. The results were similar to those found by many investigators: all of the monkeys injected for a second time with the MV strain were protected against paralysis. They were immune.

But Burnet and Macnamara took their observations one step further. They not only injected monkeys with the MV strain, but also later challenged them with a different strain, the Victoria strain, first isolated from the spinal cord of a child who had died of polio in Melbourne in 1928. This time all the monkeys got polio. Inoculation with the MV strain didn't protect against disease caused by the Victoria strain. This finding meant that there were at least two different *types* of polio virus, and infection with one type didn't protect against disease caused by another type.

The findings of Burnet and Macnamara were greeted with skepticism, but the implications were clear: if more than one type of polio virus existed, then more than one type would need to be included in a vaccine. And if there were many types, a vaccine might not be possible. The situation was analogous to that for the common cold today. Colds are caused in large part by a virus called rhinovirus. One reason that it is so difficult to make a vaccine to prevent colds is that there are at least one hundred different types of rhinoviruses.

During the next twenty years, investigators sponsored by the National Foundation worked to determine how many different types of polio viruses caused polio. Studies required thousands of monkeys and were time consuming, expensive, and tedious; investigators had to check and cross-check about two hundred strains of polio viruses sent in from all over the world. Strains submitted for testing were named for the polio victim from whom the virus had been obtained (for example, the Mahoney strain); the investigator who had isolated the virus (the Lansing strain, named for Armstrong Lansing); the group infected with the strain (the Middle Eastern Forces, or MEF, strain); or the physical characteristics of the chimpanzee used to study the virus (the Brunhilde strain, named after a female warrior in Norse

mythology). Some strains were the same type (Mahoney and Brunhilde), and some strains were different (Mahoney and Lansing). In the
end, investigators found three different types of polio viruses. Type 1
accounted for 80 percent of all cases, and types 2 and 3 each accounted
for 10 percent.

The stage was set for the development of the polio vaccine. Only one
major obstacle remained, the removal of which would lead to the only
Nobel Prize awarded to polio researchers.

Louis Pasteur's rabies vaccine, using spinal cords from rabbits,
occasionally came with a high price: permanent paralysis and death.
Now we know why. The brain and spinal cord contain myelin basic
protein, which forms a sheath around nerves similar to the rubber
sheath that surrounds an electrical wire. Pasteur's rabies vaccine, which
contained rabbit myelin basic protein, would occasionally induce an
immune response against the nervous system that caused paralysis.
Paralysis following Pasteur's vaccine was rare, occurring in about
0.4 percent of those inoculated, but researchers feared the use of monkey spinal cords to make a polio vaccine. Scientists had to find a source
of cells other than the brain or spinal cord in which to grow polio virus.

Three men solved the problem and made a practical polio vaccine
possible: John Enders, Thomas Weller, and Frederick Robbins. John
Franklin Enders was the son of John Ostrum Enders, president and
later chairman of the board of Hartford National Bank, and the grandson of the president of the Aetna Life Insurance Company. His father
left Enders an estate worth approximately $19 million. A quiet, reticent
man, Enders pursued subjects that interested him. In the mid-1940s,
Enders was interested in figuring out how to grow viruses in cells
obtained from animals. Two pediatricians pursuing graduate studies,
Thomas Weller and Frederick Robbins, assisted him.

On March 30, 1948, Thomas Weller took the arm and shoulder of
an aborted human fetus; trimmed the skin, fat, and muscle from the
arm; minced the tissues with fine scissors; and transferred them to
twelve separate flasks containing nutrient broth. Four of the flasks
were inoculated with chickenpox (varicella) virus; four, with polio
virus; and four, with no virus (to serve as a control). Because polio
virus had never been successfully grown in cells other than those obtained from nervous tissue, no one in the lab thought that Weller's

experiment would work. Fred Robbins later remembered that "one day, when Tom and I were preparing a new set of cultures, Dr. Enders suggested that, since we had some polio virus stored in the freezer, we might inoculate some of the cultures with this material, which we did. We didn't expect much."

Every few days Weller removed the nutrient fluids that bathed the fetal tissues and tested them for the presence of polio virus. To determine whether polio virus was present, nutrient fluids were injected into mice. If the mice became paralyzed, then polio virus was present. Weller found not only that the nutrient fluids paralyzed the mice, but also that the fluids could be diluted 1,000,000,000,000,000,000-fold and still cause paralysis. Clearly polio virus grew in the cells in the flasks. Later, the group found that polio virus could be grown in human foreskins (obtained by circumcisions), in human kidneys, and in monkey kidneys. They also found, when looking through a microscope, that the cells infected with polio virus appeared to shrivel and die.

The discoveries of Enders, Weller, and Robbins were important for several reasons. First, large quantities of polio virus could now be grown in cells in the laboratory (therefore, live animals would no longer be necessary to grow it). Second, the fact that polio virus could be grown in something other than nervous cell tissue relieved concerns about paralysis and death resulting from nervous tissue vaccines. Third, live polio virus could be detected quickly and inexpensively by merely looking at infected cells through a microscope (previously live virus could be detected only if it paralyzed animals).

In 1954, Enders, Weller, and Robbins received the Nobel Prize in Medicine. Characteristically, Enders refused to accept the award unless his two graduate students were included. Fred Robbins recalled: "John Enders could well have been the sole recipient, and no one would have considered it improper, including Tom Weller and me. The fact that it came about as it did is entirely due to the generosity of Dr. Enders. This attitude on the part of Enders reflected the greatness of the man." The three men split the prize money of $36,000 equally.

By 1951 Basil O'Connor had directed the National Foundation for Infantile Paralysis for thirteen years. During that time, not one child had been immunized with a polio vaccine. O'Connor watched year after year while scientists, funded with millions of dollars from his foundation, studied monkey spinal cords, inoculated mice, and stared at virus-infected cells through microscopes. No one seemed to be in a hurry to make a polio vaccine.

O'Connor didn't understand scientists. As a powerful lawyer and adviser to the president, he was used to getting what he wanted and getting it quickly. He had written many of Roosevelt's speeches, including his acceptance speech for the presidential nomination of 1932. He had also recruited Roosevelt's Brain Trust, served as a personal lawyer to the Roosevelt family, and organized Roosevelt's papers for the first presidential library. O'Connor understood men who wanted money and he understood men who wanted power, but scientists—apparently moved by neither—were harder to compel to do his bidding. They all seemed perfectly comfortable huddled in their laboratories, studying one small aspect of one small virus for the rest of their lives. They weren't in a rush to do anything. O'Connor was frustrated by their ponderous, circumspect, measured ways.

In the fall of 1951, on the thousand-foot, grandly appointed deck of the world's most elegant luxury liner, the *Queen Mary,* Basil O'Connor met a man who seemed to be different from other scientists—Jonas Salk. Both men were returning from a meeting of polio researchers at the University of Copenhagen in Denmark. O'Connor spent many hours with Salk, walking the ship's decks and sharing his philosophies about life, research, and polio. He saw in Salk a restless, kindred spirit: "Before that ship landed I knew that this was one young man to keep an eye on," said O'Connor.

Jonas Salk was born on October 28, 1914, in a tenement at 106th Street and Madison Avenue in East Harlem, New York, the first son of Russian immigrant parents and the eldest of three brothers. Jonas's two younger brothers were also successful. Herman was a veterinarian who served on UN food and health committees, and Lee was a psychologist who had gained national attention with his observation that babies were calmed by the sound of a human heart. Lee Salk's books, *What Every Child Would Like His Parents to Know* and *My Father, My Son: Intimate Relationships,* were bestsellers. In the 1970s Lee frequently appeared on the *Today Show* and *Good Morning America,* where he gave advice on child rearing.

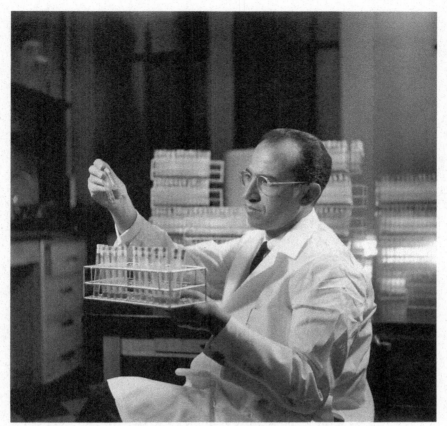

Jonas Salk, 1954 (courtesy of the March of Dimes Birth Defects Foundation).

When he was twelve years old, Jonas Salk was accepted to Townsend Harris High School in New York City, an elite, highly competitive public school. At the age of fifteen, after finishing four years of high school in three, Salk entered City College of New York and later won a scholarship to the Medical School at New York University. Following medical school, Salk was chosen from a pool of 250 applicants for an internship and residency at Mt. Sinai Hospital in New York City. Like all trainees at prestigious medical centers, he wasn't paid during his internship and received $15.00 a month during residency. The pivotal moment in Salk's career came in December 1941, after the United States entered World War II. Having just finished his medical residency, Salk was given a choice. He could either apply for a commission as a doctor in the armed forces or remain in the United States to pursue a scientific career. Salk chose science and decided to work on an influenza vaccine with Thomas Francis at the University of Michigan. Salk had no trouble proving that his work with Francis was vital to national defense: an influenza epidemic during World War I had killed forty-four thousand American soldiers. Ironically, years later, Thomas Francis would be the man to whom the National Foundation turned when it wanted to find out whether Jonas Salk's polio vaccine worked.

By 1947, Salk, now thirty-three years old with a wife, two young sons, and a wealth of experience studying viruses, decided to strike out on his own. He took a job as an associate professor at the University of Pittsburgh Medical School and director of the Virus Research Laboratory. He received support from the National Foundation in a mop-up role—that is, to confirm the work of other investigators who had found that there were three types of polio virus. Polio-typing studies were slow, tedious, repetitive, and boring, but Salk was the right man for the job. His wife, Donna, later recalled that Salk "decided one day to clean the stove. So he pulled it out from the wall, and I still have this picture in my mind of his asking for a toothpick so that he could clean out the grooves in the screws. It took him hours to do this."

To help with the polio-typing studies, Salk recruited several people to work in his laboratory. The most talented member of the team, and later the most accomplished, was Julius Youngner. Like Salk, a New Yorker and graduate of New York University, Youngner was often the primary author and creative influence behind many publications. He would later become president of the American Society for Virology and professor and chairman of the Department of Microbiology at the University of Pittsburgh. Although the loyalty of the research team members would soon be tested, they devoted themselves to the polio vaccine program. "I worked harder at that time of my life than at any time before or since," Youngner recalled.

Between 1949 and 1951 Salk injected 17,500 monkeys with 250 strains of polio virus, only to find that the previous studies were correct: there were only three types of polio virus. Although Salk's work only confirmed what was already known, his commitment and energy impressed other researchers.

In 1951 Salk received a grant from the National Foundation to develop a polio vaccine. The money—a phenomenal $200,000 per year—enabled him to expand the size and scope of his studies. Soon Salk employed more than fifty people and supervised a research laboratory that occupied three spacious, previously empty floors of Pittsburgh's Municipal Hospital, which had been built for the city by FDR's Public Works Administration. At the time that Salk received his grant, Harry Weaver was the research director of the National Foundation. Weaver recalled the following:

> There was nobody like him in those days. Perhaps one other young man was his equal as a laboratory worker, but not more than one. His approach was entirely different from that which had dominated the field. The older workers had all been brought up in the days when you didn't accept a grant of more than four or five hundred dollars from an outside source without having a long conference with the dean. Everything was on a small scale. You made do with one or two laboratory animals because you couldn't afford to pay for the twelve that were needed. Jonas had no such psychology. He thought big. He wanted lots of space, was perfectly comfortable with the idea of using hundreds of monkeys and running dozens of experiments at one time. He always wanted to expand his program so that it would encompass as much of the subject as possible. He was out of phase with the tradition of narrowing research down to one or two details, making progress inch by inch. He wanted to leap, not crawl.

But Salk's ambition incurred the wrath of other polio researchers, one of whom described his laboratory as "a big, damned industrial plant." Weaver also recognized Salk's darker side—a man rarely at peace, rarely satisfied: "No matter how well his affairs seemed to be going . . . he was always sufficiently unhappy with himself or his situation to keep driving. The harder he drove himself, the closer he came to the unattainable perfection he sought."

In 1943, while Jonas Salk was working on an influenza vaccine, there were ten thousand cases of polio in the United States; in 1948, when Salk was typing polio viruses, there were twenty-seven thousand cases of polio; in 1952, when Salk was first testing his ideas on how to make a polio vaccine, there were fifty-nine thousand cases of polio. Almost every American was directly or indirectly affected by this

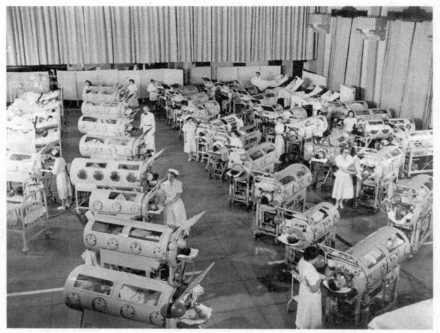

Iron lungs; Hondo, California, December 1952 (courtesy of the March of Dimes Birth Defects Foundation).

disease. A national poll conducted at the time found that polio was second only to the atomic bomb as the thing that Americans feared most. There was a desperate, growing need to prevent polio.

Between 1948 and 1952 Jonas Salk and Julius Youngner developed a series of exceptionally innovative techniques; these techniques allowed for the development of the first polio vaccine in twenty years that could be tested in people.

To develop a practical method to grow and type polio viruses, Salk and Youngner used cells from monkey testicles. Male monkeys were anesthetized and their testicles carefully removed, finely minced, and placed into glass roller tubes that were about the size of a cigar. About two hundred roller tubes could be filled with cells made from a single monkey testicle. Salk and Youngner found that polio virus grown in monkey testicular cells—like polio virus grown in monkey spinal cords—paralyzed monkeys.

Roller tubes also provided an easy method to detect polio antibodies. Previously if researchers wanted to detect antibodies, they would mix serum with virus and inject the mixture into the brains of monkeys. Now the serum-virus mixture was inoculated into the roller tubes filled with monkey testicular cells. If polio antibodies were present, cells remained alive; if not, the cells were destroyed by the virus—a phenomenon that was easily seen through the microscope. Further, by testing various dilutions of serum, Salk and Youngner could determine the amount, or titer, of polio antibodies.

Concerned that people would never accept a polio vaccine grown in monkey testicles, Salk and Youngner looked for other types of cells that supported the growth of polio virus. They tested monkey liver, kidney, and muscle cells in the roller tubes and found that kidney cells worked best. One monkey kidney provided enough cells to make between eight hundred and one thousand roller tube cultures. (Monkey kidney cells are still used today to make most polio vaccines.) Now, to grow polio virus, determine the quantity of live polio virus, and determine the titer of polio antibodies in serum, researchers could use thousands of roller tubes instead of thousands of monkeys.

Salk and Youngner had revolutionized polio virus typing. During their experiments, they learned which strains easily infected cells in roller tubes and which strains induced high titers of polio antibodies in monkeys. They used this information to pick strains for their polio vaccine. Because there were three different types of polio virus, Salk and Youngner knew that they would need to include three different strains of the virus in their vaccine. To represent type 1 polio virus, Salk chose the Mahoney strain—a decision that would haunt him for years. The Mahoney strain was isolated from a child in Akron, Ohio, whose last name was Mahoney. Although several members of the Mahoney family had live polio virus in their intestines, none had symptoms of polio. Unfortunately, infection with the Mahoney strain wasn't limited to the Mahoneys. The Klines, living next door, were also infected. Three of five Kline children were paralyzed and later died from the disease—an early clue to the unique virulence of the Mahoney strain.

The Mahoney strain had another characteristic that made it exceptionally dangerous. Although virtually all strains of polio virus paralyzed monkeys after injection into their brains or spinal cords, only a few strains paralyzed them after injection into their muscles—the route by which children would soon be inoculated. Not only did undiluted preparations of the Mahoney strain paralyze monkeys after injection into their muscles, but it also paralyzed them after the preparation was diluted 1 to 10, 1 to 100, 1 to 1,000, and 1 to 10,000 in salt water. The incredible virulence of the Mahoney strain was based on the fact that after injection into muscles, it was ten thousand times more likely to enter the bloodstream and travel to the brain and spinal cord than any other polio strain. Salk knew that 80 percent of all polio infections were caused by type 1 viruses. By choosing the Mahoney strain, he had picked the most virulent strain from the most virulent type of virus. If he didn't successfully kill all of the polio virus particles that were present in his vaccine—a vaccine that would soon be inoculated into the muscles of hundreds of thousands of children—he risked causing paralysis. In part, Salk picked the Mahoney strain because of its virulence. He reasoned that because very small quantities of Mahoney virus caused paralysis in monkeys, researchers would easily detect residual live virus inadvertently contained in the vaccine. If Salk had picked a weaker type 1 strain (such as the Brunhilde), the risk of paralysis would have been much smaller. However, the vaccine might have been much less effective. Two years later, in front of a congressional hearing, Albert Sabin, a polio researcher who later developed his own polio vaccine, said, in reference to the Mahoney strain, that "no vaccine should be made with this dangerous virus in it."

The other two strains of virus in Salk's vaccine were not controversial. To represent type 2 virus, Salk picked the MEF-1 strain, which had been isolated from an adult who had contracted severe polio while serving in the Middle Eastern Forces in Cairo, Egypt, during World War II. To represent type 3 virus, Salk picked a strain that was isolated from a boy named James Sarkett. Unfortunately, the label on the specimen collected from the boy was written sloppily, and the "r" was mistaken for a "u." As a result, the strain has always been referred to in scientific presentations, medical journals, and product inserts as the Saukett strain.

To make his vaccine, Salk took the three strains of polio virus grown in monkey kidney or testicular cells, placed the virus suspensions on melting ice, and, just like Maurice Brodie before him, treated the virus with formaldehyde. During the inactivation process, Salk periodically took the mixture out of the tubes, injected it into the brains of monkeys, and waited to see if the monkeys were paralyzed. Depending on the strain, he found that the mixture no longer paralyzed monkeys after about ten days of formaldehyde treatment. To make sure that polio virus was completely killed, Salk treated the virus with formaldehyde for another one to two days. The strain of virus that took the longest time to kill was Mahoney.

The D. T. Watson Home, where Salk performed his first vaccine studies, was originally the home of David T. Watson, a prominent Pittsburgh lawyer who was ambassador to England in the early 1900s. During his visits to England and Switzerland, Watson had visited sanitaria that gave victims of tuberculosis a clean, open-air environment in which to heal. Watson and his wife willed that their country estate in the wealthy suburb of Sewickley Heights, twelve miles northwest of Pittsburgh, be used as a "home for destitute poor white female children between the ages of three and sixteen years, especially including and preferring children crippled or deformed." In 1920 the D. T. Watson Home for Crippled Children opened its doors. A large brick building surrounded by manicured lawns, the Watson Home had about 120 beds and was by the mid-1950s a premier facility for taking care of girls and boys with polio.

The polio vaccine that Salk first tested in the Watson Home was actually many different vaccines. Children received a vaccine that contained either types 1, 2, or 3 polio viruses or all three types combined; a vaccine that was treated with formaldehyde for ten days or for longer; a vaccine that was grown in monkey testicular cells or in monkey kidney cells; or a vaccine that was injected just under the skin or directly into the muscles. After injecting children with these vaccines, Salk couldn't sleep. "He came back again that first night to make sure that everyone was all right," recalled Lucile Cochran, nurse superintendent at the Watson Home. "Everyone was."

Salk was fishing. He was trying to figure out which preparation looked the most promising and then perfect it. During the next few months, Salk inoculated about one hundred children at the Watson Home with different preparations of his vaccine. The results were disappointing. He found that only one of his vaccines induced polio antibodies—the vaccine that contained type 2 virus. Vaccines that contained types 1 or 3 virus did not induce any polio antibodies.

In May 1952 Salk began inoculating residents of the Polk State School, which housed mentally retarded boys and men and was about eighty miles from Pittsburgh, with a vaccine that contained all three types of polio virus. Unlike the children at the Watson Home, all of the Polk residents were inoculated with a vaccine that was suspended in mineral oil, and all were inoculated in their muscles. The mineral oil vaccine worked well: Polk residents developed antibodies to all three types of polio virus. (Mineral oil caused polio vaccine to remain in the muscles for a long time, allowing for continuous stimulation of the immune system and longer immunity. Agents, like mineral oil, that enhance immune responses are called adjuvants. Adjuvants other than mineral oil are still used in vaccines today.)

Although repugnant by today's standards, Salk's decision to inoculate retarded children with his vaccine wasn't unusual. While Salk was studying retarded children at the Polk School, studies were being performed at an institution called the Willowbrook State School that later made the gentle word Willowbrook synonymous with cruel and unethical medical experiments.

In 1938 the New York state legislature purchased 375 acres of land in the town of Willowbrook on Staten Island and authorized the construction of a facility to care for three thousand mentally retarded children. The Willowbrook State School opened its doors four years later. Its residents were "the most severely retarded, the most handicapped, and the most helpless of those being cared for in the New York State system." By 1957 more than six thousand children were packed into Willowbrook. "The overcrowded conditions in the buildings make care, treatment, supervision, and possible training of the patients difficult, if not impossible," said Jack Hammond, director of Willowbrook. "When the patients are up and in the day rooms, they are crowded together, soiling, attacking each other, abusing themselves and destroying their clothing. At night, in many of the dormitories, the beds must be placed together in order to provide sufficient space for all patients. Therefore, except for one narrow aisle, it is virtually necessary to climb over beds in order to reach the children." Faced with intolerable living conditions, Hammond sent a questionnaire to all parents that included the following option: "I wish to discuss the possibility and advisability of removing my child from Willowbrook State School." In response to this questionnaire, two children were taken home.

The overcrowding, poor sanitation, and small staff at Willowbrook fostered the spread of many infectious diseases, including hepatitis, an infection of the liver. In an effort to control outbreaks of hepatitis, school administrators asked Saul Krugman, an infectious disease specialist at Bellevue Hospital in New York City, to find a way to prevent or treat the disease. Krugman found that nine of every ten children admitted to Willowbrook developed hepatitis soon after arrival. Although it was known that hepatitis was caused by a virus, it was not known how hepatitis was spread, whether it could be prevented, or how many different types of viruses caused it. Krugman used the children of Willowbrook to answer these questions. Some of his studies involved feeding hepatitis virus to children who didn't have the disease. In 1957 about sixty retarded children between three and ten years of age were fed hepatitis virus prepared from the feces of children known to have the disease, and Krugman watched during the next few weeks as they developed fever, nausea, vomiting, intolerance to food, jaundice (a yellowing of the skin and eyes), and liver damage.

During his studies at Willowbrook, Krugman learned a lot about hepatitis virus. He identified two different types, A and B. He showed how the viruses were transmitted. And he demonstrated that gamma globulin, a preparation of serum taken from people who had recovered from hepatitis, protected against disease. Mankind clearly benefited from Saul Krugman's studies. Krugman reasoned that the prevention of serious and fatal hepatitis in many outweighed causing transient hepatitis in a few. But looking through the window of current standards, many consider Krugman's studies to be highly unethical.

Salk showed that polio virus grown in his laboratory, inactivated with formaldehyde, suspended in mineral oil, and injected into children induced polio antibodies in blood and serum. During the studies at Watson and Polk, Salk spent many hours looking through the microscope at cells inoculated with mixtures of viruses and children's serum.

He saw that cells were protected even after the sera were diluted many times. "It was the thrill of my life," remembered Salk. "Compared to the feeling I got seeing those results under the microscope, everything that followed was anti-climactic." And the vaccine was safe. There were no signs of illness that could be attributed to the vaccine. "I've got it," he said to his wife.

But Salk knew that he had a long road ahead. "Although the results obtained in these studies can be regarded as encouraging," he said, "they should not be interpreted to indicate that a practical vaccine is now at hand."

On January 23, 1953, Jonas Salk presented his findings at a meeting of the National Foundation for Infantile Paralysis in Hershey, Pennsylvania. Those in attendance were impressed with his progress; they thought that Salk's mineral oil vaccine could be the one to protect children against polio. Joe Smadel, scientific director of the Walter Reed Army Medical Center in Washington, D.C., was ready to push forward with a large-scale trial of Salk's vaccine in hundreds of thousands of children: "What are you waiting for?" Smadel asked. "Why don't you get ready and put on a proper field trial?" But Salk wasn't ready. He pleaded for more time to make a better vaccine.

Although Salk kept his studies at Watson and Polk a secret, the results were leaked to the press. A nationally syndicated column carried the headline "New Polio Vaccine—Big Hopes Seen," and on February 9, 1953, an article appeared in *Time* magazine next to Salk's picture, claiming that "there was solid good news on the polio front last week." But Salk worried that he didn't have a vaccine and that the press would only agitate a nation desperate for one. He feared that the less time he had to develop a vaccine, the less effective the vaccine would be. And he knew that on March 28, 1953, a paper reporting his findings at Watson and Polk would be published in the *Journal of the American Medical Association*. He wanted to lower public expectations. So he went to Basil O'Connor and asked to speak directly to the American public.

At 10:45 P.M. on March 26, 1953, two days before the publication of his studies at Watson and Polk, Jonas Salk appeared on the CBS national radio program *The Scientist Speaks for Himself*. After a lengthy introduction describing the history of polio, Salk continued: "In the studies that are being reported this week, it has also been shown that the amount of antibody induced by vaccination compares favorably with that which develops after natural infection. The results of these studies provide justification for optimism, and it does appear that the approach in these investigations may lead to the desired objective. *But this has not yet been accomplished.*"

The response to the program was predictable. Salk became the embodiment of a vaccine that would soon save the world from polio. To the public, he was an immediate hero. But members of the scientific community criticized Salk for talking about unpublished data and for pandering to the media. The radio address marked the beginning of an animosity that Salk would suffer for the rest of his life. One critic said, "What adult would be naïve enough to think that he could go on radio and television to talk about a polio vaccine he was making and expect to be allowed to retreat to his cloister afterward? Naïve, my foot. Whether he believes it or not, Jonas went on the air that night to take a bow and become a public hero. And that's what he became." During the next few years, the jealousy, anger, and hostility toward Salk would get in the way of his science and limit his ability to convince his colleagues of the real value of his vaccine.

In the spring of 1953 Jonas Salk performed the time-honored rite of vaccinating himself, his wife Donna, and his three children (Peter, age nine; Darrell, age six; and Jonathan, age three) with his mineral oil vaccine. Salk believed in his vaccine: "It is courage based on confidence, not daring," he said. "Our kids were lined up to get the vaccine," recalled Donna Salk. "I remember taking it for granted. I had complete and utter confidence in Jonas."

Salk believed that one dose of his mineral oil vaccine would protect children against polio. Thomas Rivers, the director of vaccine research for the National Foundation, agreed and would have pushed forward with Salk's vaccine if it hadn't been for one man—Joseph Bell. An epidemiologist at the National Institutes of Health, Bell was recruited by the National Foundation to design the test of Salk's vaccine. Bell believed that mineral oil wasn't safe for children because in his experience, people occasionally developed "painful arms and running abscesses that took months to heal." When the National Foundation received Bell's report, it decided against using a mineral oil vaccine.

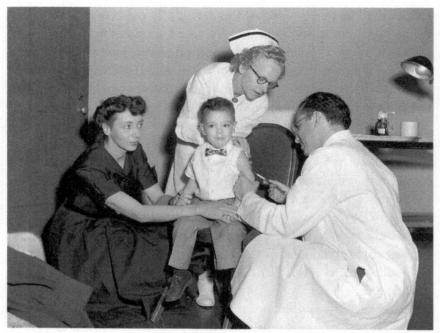

Jonas Salk inoculates son Jonathan; May 16, 1953 (courtesy of the March of Dimes Birth Defects Foundation).

Now it was up to Salk to make a vaccine knowing that his studies without mineral oil were very discouraging and that only one preparation without mineral oil had worked. "All we had was a flicker of light," said Salk. Between March and October 1953 Salk performed a series of unprecedented studies that remain unmatched. He figured out a method to make a vaccine without mineral oil and at the same time formulated what was to become a controversial mathematical model to ensure the vaccine's safety. He conducted these studies under tremendous pressure from the press, the National Foundation, and a public that every day heard the drumbeat of children paralyzed by polio.

To create a polio vaccine without mineral oil, Salk proposed three changes. He made the new vaccine using monkey kidney cells (monkey testicular cells were out); less formaldehyde (formaldehyde was now diluted 1 to 4,000 instead of 1 to 250); and higher temperatures during inactivation (98 degrees Fahrenheit instead of 33 degrees). To ensure that the vaccine was safe, Salk injected it into the brains of monkeys and onto cells in roller tubes. Both the monkeys and the cells remained healthy. Because he knew that the vaccine would soon be given to hundreds of thousands of children in a large field trial, Salk had to find a method that ensured the absence of even one infectious virus particle in hundreds of thousands of doses. So he devised his "straight-line" theory of inactivation, which defined the relationship between the quantity of infectious virus and the length of time that the virus was treated with formaldehyde. The theory was at the heart of the tragedy that would soon follow.

Salk's straight-line theory of inactivation is explained as follows: the volume of one dose of vaccine given to children at Watson and Polk was one milliliter—roughly one-half of a thimbleful of fluid. Salk showed that before treatment with formaldehyde one dose contained about 1 million infectious virus particles. Treatment with formaldehyde caused the quantity of virus to decrease steadily and predictably. After treatment for twelve hours, one dose contained 100,000 infectious virus particles; after treatment for twenty-four hours, only 10,000; after treatment for seventy-two hours, only one infectious particle remained—the other 999,999 had been killed by formaldehyde. The quantity of live polio virus in the vaccine had been reduced one millionfold in three days.

When Salk plotted the quantity of virus against the length of time that virus was treated with formaldehyde, the points connected in a straight line. Salk reasoned that if the virus was treated for three more days and the line remained straight, then another millionfold reduction would occur. Thus instead of one infectious particle in one dose, there should be one infectious particle in 1 million doses. Treatment for another three days should reduce the quantity of live virus to one infectious virus in 1 trillion doses—more vaccine than would be necessary to vaccinate the entire world. For all practical purposes, treatment for nine days would completely inactivate polio virus.

The graph Salk constructed consisted of two parts: a part a researcher could test in a laboratory and a part that one assumed to be true. It was possible to test virus preparations and find that they contained one to 1 million infectious particles in one dose (the "fact" part of the graph), but it was not practical to test 1 million to 1 trillion doses

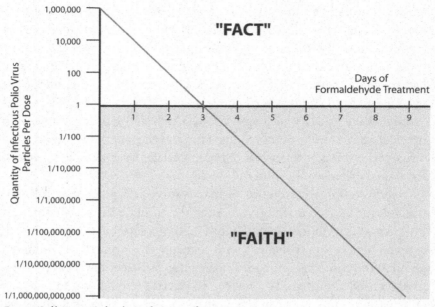

Jonas Salk's straight-line theory of inactivation.

to find that they contained one infectious particle (the "faith" part of the graph). So the extrapolation from the quantities of virus found during the first few days of inactivation to the quantities found after nine days of inactivation was a matter of believing that the line remained straight. If instead the line curved back toward the baseline, then live virus might still be present. For several years after the events that occurred in the spring of 1955, Jonas Salk was the only scientist in America or Europe who believed that the line remained straight.

Eight months after Salk published his studies of children given inactivated polio vaccine, two prominent researchers had difficulties reproducing his findings. On November 10, 1953, at a meeting of the American Public Health Association in New York City, Albert Milzer of the Michael Reese Hospital in Chicago stated, "We followed very rigidly the conditions of [formaldehyde] inactivation as outlined by Salk. For reasons not apparent to us we were not successful in consistently completely inactivating the virus." Using Salk's technique, Milzer showed that live polio virus was still present and capable of paralyzing monkeys even after treatment with formaldehyde. Milzer warned: "Before undertaking a field study to evaluate a poliomyelitis vaccine we feel that it would be advisable to proceed cautiously . . . for we must avoid the tragic consequences that have accompanied poliomyelitis vaccine research in the past." Salk was furious. Writing to a friend, he said, "These investigators have, without justification, impugned experiments that were carefully conducted and they have aroused fear and doubt by their irresponsible remarks in a scientific paper in which evidence rather than opinion should stand out."

Ten months after Milzer's warnings, on September 8, 1954, Salk presented his inactivation data to an international audience of polio researchers in Rome. At the end of the presentation, Sven Gard, a highly regarded virologist at the Karolinska Institute in Stockholm and member of the Nobel Prize Committee, said, "We have studied the effect of formaldehyde on poliomyelitis virus, [and] in our hands, the inactivation does not run the course of a [straight-line] reaction. . . . To obtain the safety margin set by Dr. Salk . . . we would have to extend our formaldehyde treatment for 12 weeks." In other words, Gard did not agree with Salk's straight-line theory. Rather, he found that as polio virus was treated with formaldehyde for longer and longer intervals, the line started to curve. Salk fully inactivated virus in nine days; Gard, in twelve weeks. Gard ended his presentation with the following statement: "I just wanted to report these observations, as I think they have a bearing on the problem of production of a safe and effective field vaccine."

While Sven Gard was warning researchers in Rome of a possible problem with Salk's inactivation methods, four hundred thousand American children were receiving Salk's vaccine.

The Grand Experiment

There is always the possibility of human error.
—Jonas Salk, 1954

IN THE FALL OF 1953, THE NATIONAL FOUNDA-
tion for Infantile Paralysis wanted to perform a large trial of Jonas Salk's vaccine. Unfortunately, Salk didn't have a vaccine. But he was getting close.

In 1952 the United States had suffered its worst polio epidemic; fifty-eight thousand people (or one of every three thousand Americans) had been affected. To determine whether Salk's vaccine could prevent a disease that occurred in roughly 0.03 percent of the population, hundreds of thousands of children would need to be immunized. Only pharmaceutical companies had the facilities and resources to make that much vaccine, so that was where the National Foundation turned.

The first pharmaceutical company approached by the foundation, Parke-Davis, of Detroit, Michigan, had experience making vaccines and had scientists, like Fred Stimpert, who had worked with polio virus. Impressed with the company's expertise, the foundation granted Parke-Davis exclusive rights to make polio vaccine for the trial, tentatively scheduled to begin in eight months.

Parke-Davis first had to develop a detailed manufacturing protocol. Because Salk was still working on his vaccine, he didn't have a protocol. "We needed adequate commercial product by the end of 1953 and could not achieve it unless I worked closely with Parke-Davis laboratory, and vice-versa," said Salk. "I had still not had time to advance my work to the point of deciding which combination of virus, [formaldehyde], temperature, inactivation time, acidity, and so on would yield a vaccine most suitable for the field trial, yet here I found myself to all intents and purposes committed by [the National Foundation] to assist in the manufacturing process. Naturally, the expected took place. The Parke-Davis people were interested in 'product.' Since I had none, but had only a set of principles on which more work was needed, they concluded that they might be able to develop a vaccine on their own before I could develop mine."

Parke-Davis in turn became increasingly frustrated with Salk—they didn't believe that he knew what he was doing. "Besides the technical problems they were having with Jonas's process, the Parke-Davis scientists were pessimistic about what he was driving at," one foundation official remembered. "They didn't think Jonas was far enough advanced in his own research to justify all the tooling-up they were doing. I remember one New York conference at which one of them actually questioned Jonas, got answers that did not satisfy him and said, straight out, 'Jonas does not have a vaccine.'" Parke-Davis also had other motives. They had already patented a different method to inactivate viruses—ultraviolet irradiation. If Parke-Davis used ultraviolet irradiation to inactivate polio virus, they could exclude other companies from competition.

As the relationship with Parke-Davis soured, Salk urged the National Foundation to encourage other pharmaceutical companies to make his vaccine. In November 1953 O'Connor met with top executives of several companies in New York City; by February 1954, four more had agreed to participate: Eli Lilly of Indianapolis, Indiana; Wyeth Laboratories of Marietta, Pennsylvania; Pitman-Moore of Zionville, Indiana; and Cutter Laboratories of Berkeley, California.

To entice companies to make vaccine for the field trial, O'Connor made an unusual offer: he would buy 27 million doses of vaccine at a cost of $9 million. O'Connor didn't offer to buy vaccine for the field trial (companies were expected to pay for that themselves); rather, he offered to buy all the vaccine after the trial was over. O'Connor was gambling that the field trial would show that the vaccine worked. But even if it didn't work and wasn't later sold, companies would still be paid. Basil O'Connor and the National Foundation had taken the risk out of vaccine research and development.

Thus by early 1954 five companies had lined up to make vaccine for

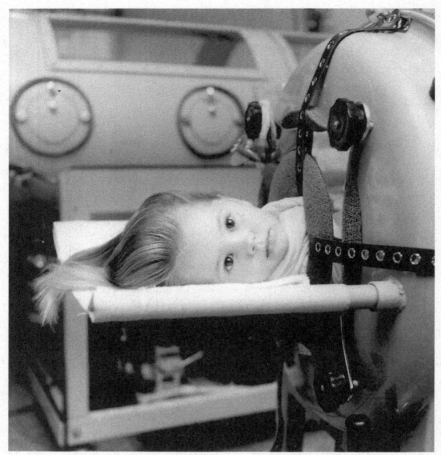

Regina Edwards; Houston, Texas, July 1952. Many children in iron lungs died from pneumonia (courtesy of the March of Dimes Birth Defects Foundation).

the field trial, but Salk still hesitated to provide a detailed protocol to the manufacturers. Before the field trial, Salk had published a paper that stated "the precise details of the methods which have been developed for destroying the infectivity of polio virus by formaldehyde . . . as yet have not been published. A fuller presentation and documentation of details here referred to will be covered in several reports to be made in the appropriate technical journals." But Salk never published those details.

Why was Jonas Salk hesitant to provide specific instructions to manufacturers on how to make his vaccine? Certainly he knew what was at stake; the National Foundation was about to inoculate hundreds of thousands of children. The reason for Salk's hesitation is found in several papers published prior to the field trial, where Salk talked at great length about his concepts of inactivation, his straight-line theory, the importance of filtration before inactivation, and how large and small batches of polio virus might have different rates of inactivation. Salk believed that if pharmaceutical company scientists understood his theories, the details of manufacture were unimportant. He described the inactivation of virus as an art: "The method is very much like the one a housewife uses when she wants to prepare a new dessert, say a cake. She starts with an idea and certain ingredients, and then experiments, a little more of this and a little less of that, and keeps changing things until finally she has a good recipe. In the process, she will have deduced certain universal laws which govern such things. From there, she can go on to make further improvements during the years."

By February 1, 1954, Jonas Salk had developed a fifty-five-page protocol for the manufacture of polio vaccine. The second appendix included a thorough description of Salk's concept of straight-line inactivation and a recommendation that at least four samples of formaldehyde-treated virus be collected during the inactivation process. But many details—such as the type of filter to be used prior to inactivation, the maximum quantity of virus to be inactivated, and the exact intervals during inactivation when samples should be tested—were not included. By omitting such specific details, Salk had challenged the manufacturers to find a protocol that worked for each of them; they had to adapt Salk's straight-line concept of inactivation to conditions in their plants; it didn't matter how they did it. Not all companies welcomed the challenge. One scientist at Cutter Laboratories wrote to a friend that "the name Salk is a dirty word around here." Another said "every batch is a damned research project."

Companies competed for months to be the first to make the most vaccine for the field trial. The winners, not surprisingly, were those with the most experience making vaccines—Parke-Davis and Eli Lilly. Cutter Laboratories had a harder time than the others. Two lots of vaccine made by Cutter didn't contain all three types of polio virus—type 2 was mistakenly omitted. No other company committed this error.

Joseph Bell, the man responsible for steering the National Foundation away from Salk's mineral oil vaccine, was now responsible for determining the size and scope of the field trial. Bell decided that samples of every batch, or lot, of vaccine that was given to children should first be tested for safety by three groups: the manufacturer, Jonas Salk, and the National Institutes of Health. The last group was included because it would eventually be responsible for licensing the vaccine. The specific group within the National Institutes for Health responsible for licensing vaccines was the Laboratory of Biologics Control. (Although vaccines were first used in the United States in the early 1800s [Jenner's smallpox vaccine], the regulation of vaccines was still in its infancy. Scientists at the Laboratory of Biologics Control spent most of their time doing research that had little to do with the vaccines that they regulated; vaccine regulation was more like a hobby than a full-time job.)

The trial of Salk's vaccine was in serious trouble before it started. Four of the first six lots of formaldehyde-inactivated vaccine made by Parke-Davis and Eli Lilly contained live polio virus. The problem was first noted by the head of the Laboratory of Biologics Control, William Workman. A pleasant, shy man with a shock of gray hair, Workman had spent most of his life working as a scientist for the federal government. When Workman saw that companies were having trouble reproducing Salk's methods, he immediately sent a letter to Salk asking that the field trial be postponed. The letter was written on March 22, 1954, only weeks before the trial was scheduled to begin. Workman was worried not only because he had found live virus in certain lots of the vaccine made by Lilly and Parke-Davis, but also because he feared that live virus might be present in other lots that had passed safety tests. "Under the circumstances, I cannot escape the feeling that an occasional lot . . . which does pass the test may actually contain living virus and be unsafe for use," wrote Workman. "My recommendation is that the proposed field studies be postponed until—(1) specifications and minimum requirements can be revised to give greater assurance of the safety of the final product; (2) it has been shown that the vaccine prepared in accordance with such specifications meets acceptable criteria for safety."

Workman's letter precipitated a tense meeting that included O'Connor; Thomas Rivers, the chief scientific adviser to the National Foundation; James Shannon, assistant director of the National Institutes of Health; and Victor Haas, director of the National Microbiological Institute, within the National Institutes of Health. Shannon was Haas's boss, and Haas was Workman's boss. Rivers recalled the meeting: "I will tell you plainly that Dr. James Shannon and Dr. Victor Haas of the U.S. Public Health Service at that time were against passing the vaccine. As a matter of fact, Dr. Haas said that in his view the vaccine was dangerous and that he would not give it to his own children."

On March 25, 1954, after heated negotiations, the field trial was allowed to proceed with one condition: companies had to make eleven consecutive lots of vaccine that passed safety tests before their manufacturing methods could be accepted with confidence.

But the field trial suffered one more setback before it began. Walter Winchell, a journalist whose column was syndicated in more than two thousand newspapers and whose radio program at its peak reached 55 million Americans, found out about the problems at Eli Lilly and Parke-Davis. The inventor of the gossip column, Winchell had launched his career on the sentiment that "the way to become famous is to throw a brick at someone who is famous." On April 4, 1954, Winchell began his radio program with his signature opening: "Good evening, Mr. and Mrs. America and all the friends at sea. Attention everyone! In a few moments I will report on a new polio vaccine—it may be a killer!" Winchell's staccato delivery coupled with his ability to speak 240 words per minute made for a broadcast that sounded like machine gun fire. Following a commercial break, he continued: "Attention all doctors and families: the National Foundation for Infantile Paralysis plans to inoculate one million children with a new vaccine this month. . . . The United States Public Health Service tested ten batches of this new vaccine. . . . They found, I am told, that seven of the ten contained live, not dead, poliovirus . . . [and] that it killed several monkeys. The name of the vaccine is the Salk vaccine, named for Dr. Jonas Salk of the University of Pittsburgh." One week later, Winchell followed up his show with the statement that the National Foundation

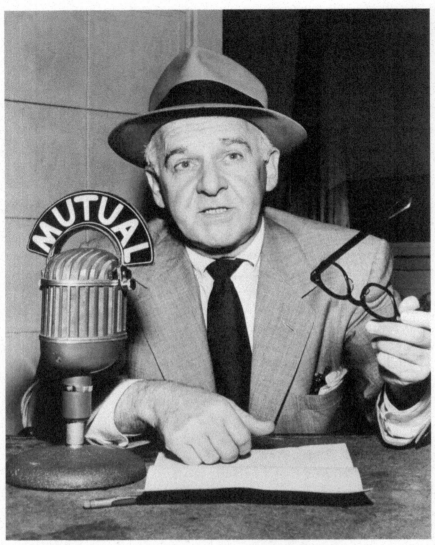

Walter Winchell at the microphone, 1955 (courtesy of the Bettmann Archives).

was stockpiling "little white coffins" in anticipation of what might occur during the field trial. Winchell said that he received his information from a "famous name held by request" who was a "former research director of the National Foundation for Infantile Paralysis who had recently been relieved of his duties." The source of the leak was Paul de Kruif. Because of Winchell's broadcast, one hundred fifty thousand children withdrew from the trial.

In the fall of 1953, Joseph Bell recommended that children should receive either a shot of Salk's polio vaccine or a shot of influenza vaccine. Bell reasoned that children who didn't receive the polio vaccine would at least receive something from which they would benefit. Vials of vaccine would be coded, and neither the nurse who was giving the shot nor the child who was getting it would know what was given.

Salk didn't agree with Bell's proposal and suggested that children should receive polio vaccine or nothing; he couldn't accept that children would think they were getting a shot of his vaccine when they weren't. In the midst of these arguments, Joseph Bell resigned.

The trial of Jonas Salk's polio vaccine now had no director and no clear plan. In December 1953, the National Foundation asked Thomas Francis, Salk's former mentor and the developer of the influenza vaccine, to direct the trial. Francis, the son of a Methodist minister, was tough, meticulous, and uncompromising. He didn't agree with Salk that children should receive either polio vaccine or nothing. Francis believed that the best way to determine whether the vaccine worked and whether it was safe was to inoculate children with either Salk's vaccine or with the fluid in which Salk's vaccine was suspended (placebo). (Ironically, the word "placebo," derived from the Latin *placere,* means "I shall please." Placebo medications, such as sugar pills, were often given for psychological rather than physiological benefit.) But Salk knew that children given placebo would be far more likely to be paralyzed or die from polio than those who received his vaccine. "What moral justification can there be for intentionally injecting children with salt solution or some other placebo?" he said. "I would feel that every child who is injected with a placebo and becomes paralyzed will do so at my hands."

After much debate, the field trial included 420,000 children injected with Salk's vaccine (made by Parke-Davis and Eli Lilly); 200,000 injected with a placebo; and 1.2 million given nothing—a total of about 1.8 million participants. On Monday, April 26, 1954, at 9:00 A.M., six-year-old Randy Kerr of McLean, Virginia, received the first shot. Smiling for the reporters and cameramen, Randy proudly announced that the shot "hurt less than a shot of penicillin." Neither Randy, his parents, nor the nurse administering the shot knew what he was getting.

The field trial supported by the National Foundation was then, and remains today, the largest, most comprehensive test of a medical product ever performed: twenty thousand physicians and health officers, forty thousand registered nurses, fourteen thousand school principals, fifty thousand teachers, and two hundred thousand citizens in forty-four states volunteered to participate. Vaccine or placebo was given to first, second, and third graders within five weeks as a series of three shots; shots were given in the back of the left arm, in the triceps muscle. Children who participated in the study received a lollipop, a pin that read "Polio Pioneer," and a chance to avoid the crippling effects of polio. (The trial, which cost $7.5 million, would cost about $5 billion today.)

The results of the trial were clear: Sixteen children in the study died from polio; none of them had received Salk's vaccine. Thirty-six children developed severe polio and had to be placed in iron lungs; only two of the thirty-six had received Salk's vaccine. Finally, children who did not receive Salk's vaccine were 3.3 times more likely to be paralyzed than those who did receive it.

The vaccine worked. But was it safe? By including a group of children injected with vaccine and a group not injected with anything, investigators knew immediately whether the vaccine was causing paralysis. Although several cases of polio occurred within two months of vaccination, Thomas Francis concluded that Salk's vaccine was not causing paralysis: "The small number of cases in vaccinated persons, the lack of correlation between site of paralysis and inoculation, the absence of association in time between vaccination and prevalence, the absence of any extension in families or in uninoculated persons in the same schoolroom, lead uniformly to this conclusion," he said.

Salk, Rivers, O'Connor, and advisers to the National Foundation

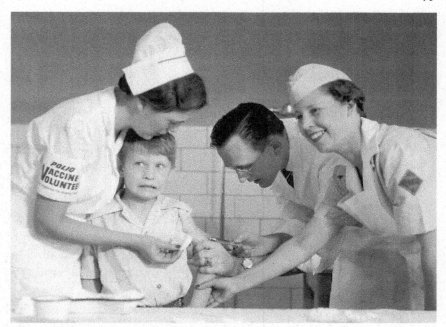

Dr. Richard Mulvaney inoculates child for field trial; McLean, Virginia, April 26, 1954 (courtesy of the March of Dimes Birth Defects Foundation).

had heard Albert Milzer and Sven Gard say that they couldn't completely inactivate polio virus using Salk's technique; they heard that four of the first six lots of vaccine produced by Parke-Davis and Eli Lilly contained live polio virus; they heard William Workman say that laboratory tests to detect live polio virus in the vaccine might be inadequate; they heard Victor Haas say that he wouldn't give the vaccine to his children; and they heard Walter Winchell proclaim to the nation that the government was making "little white coffins" to prepare for a vaccine that might be "a killer." Now 420,000 children had been given Salk's vaccine, and not one case of paralysis was apparently caused by the vaccine. Everyone involved in the planning and testing of the polio vaccine felt complete and utter relief.

With victory in hand, Thomas Francis planned to announce the results of the field trial to the press and to the public in Ann Arbor, Michigan, at the site of his Vaccine Evaluation Center. Salk, who was asked to speak, said, "I actually thought I'd go to that meeting, hear the report, read a paper of my own, talk to a few newsmen, and return to Pittsburgh and my laboratory the next day." Salk hadn't anticipated what awaited him in Ann Arbor.

On May 31, 1954, a Gallup poll showed that more Americans knew about the field trial of Jonas Salk's polio vaccine than knew the full name of the president of the United States, Dwight David Eisenhower. This was because more Americans had participated in the funding, development, and testing of the polio vaccine than had participated in the nomination and election of the president.

Thomas Francis was given the difficult task of evaluating data on 1.8 million children while trying to keep the results secret; he wanted to make sure that he recorded and analyzed every piece of information before talking to the press and the public. More than 100 million Americans sent their dimes to the National Foundation, and at least 7 million worked closely with the foundation as fund-raisers, committee workers, and volunteers at clinics and record centers. All were intensely interested in the results of Francis's study. One observer recalled that "neither [Francis] nor anyone else had ever before had the experience of analyzing some 144,000,000 bits of information involving 1,800,000 persons while the public was looking, or at least trying to look, over his shoulder to see how the data added up. It was a little like an advanced mathematics student trying to do his homework at Forty-Second and Broadway at 5:00 P.M."

In the early morning hours of April 8, 1955, Thomas Francis finished writing his report. Four days later, on April 12, at 10:20 A.M.—ten years to the day after the death of polio's most famous victim, Franklin Delano Roosevelt—Francis stepped to the podium at Rackham Hall on the campus of the University of Michigan. An elegant, salmon-colored building, Rackham Hall had a large auditorium on the first floor. Five hundred people, including 150 press, radio, and television reporters, filled the room; 16 television and newsreel cameras stood on a long platform at the back; and 54,000 physicians, sitting in movie theaters across the country, watched the broadcast on closed-circuit television. Eli Lilly paid $250,000 to broadcast the event. Americans turned on their radios to hear the details, department stores set up loudspeakers, and judges suspended trials so that everyone in the courtroom could hear what Thomas Francis was about to say. Europeans listened on the *Voice of America*.

The setting for the announcement was unusual. Typically scientists presented data in the calm, sterile, gray environment of scientific meetings, not the highly charged, brightly lit, theatrical atmosphere of Rackham Hall. "We were flabbergasted," said a member of the National Foundation. "We wanted the meeting at the National Academy of Sciences so the occasion would be as grave and solemn as any scientist could wish—and here the Michigan people were building a platform for television cameras right in the meeting room.... One thing is certain, I suppose: Even if the cameramen had been barred from the hall they would have stampeded around outside it. As O'Connor used to say, 'If Tommy [Francis] were to announce his findings in a men's room, the reporters and cameramen would be there. This thing is bigger than us all.'" A veteran newsman from the Associated Press agreed: "It wouldn't have made a particle of difference if Dr. Francis had read the report to himself in his bedroom or sent it in to the most obscure medical journal he could find. Reporters would have broken into his bedroom or stormed the journal's printing plant and taken the report out of there line by line. The Francis report was the story of the year."

Before Francis presented his data, copies of the report were brought in for the press. "They brought the report in on dollies, and newsmen were jumping over each other and screaming, 'It works! It works! It works!'" one reporter remembered. "The whole place was bedlam. One of the doctors [had] tears in his eyes."

For one hour and thirty-eight minutes Thomas Francis stood in front of the audience at Rackham Hall. Using an overhead projector, Francis worked his way through a dense thicket of charts, figures, graphs, and tables, using phrases such as "serologic testing," "antigenic potency," and "virus isolation." The presentation was numbing, but the results were clear: the vaccine worked. Inside the auditorium Francis finished to restrained applause. Outside the auditorium Americans tearfully and joyfully embraced the results. By the time Thomas Francis stepped down, church bells were ringing across the country, factories were observing moments of silence, synagogues and churches were holding prayer meetings, and parents and teachers were weeping.

One shopkeeper hung a banner on his window: *Thank you, Dr. Salk.* "It was as if a war had ended," one observer recalled.

Several others spoke at Rackham Hall that day: Alan Gregg, vice president of the Rockefeller Foundation; Basil O'Connor, director of the National Foundation; and Thomas Rivers, chairman of the Vaccine Advisory Committee of the National Foundation. All delivered brief, moving statements. When Jonas Salk rose to speak, Harry Stambaugh, president of the Watson Home, stood up, applauding. Immediately the rest of the audience rose to join the ovation. Salk stepped to the podium.

Jonas Salk was to the public the embodiment of a decades-long effort to eliminate the horror of polio. Like Lou Gehrig before him ("Today I consider myself the luckiest man on the face of this earth") or Neil Armstrong after him ("One small step for man, one giant leap for mankind"), Salk could have offered a few emotional, poignant sentences about polio and its conquest. But Salk was disappointed with the results of the field trial. He knew that his vaccine could be improved, and he saw this meeting as an opportunity to present a lengthy discussion of how, with the right modifications, his vaccine could induce even greater quantities of polio antibodies and life-long immunity. Angered by his presentation, Thomas Francis confronted Salk. "After Jonas was through talking, I went over to him, sore," said Francis. " 'What the hell did you have to say that for?' I said. 'You're in no position to claim 100 percent effectiveness. What's the matter with you?' " Salk's presentation also infuriated Thomas Rivers. "This was supposed to be Tommy Francis' day," said Rivers. "Salk should have kept his mouth shut. Tommy had reported on the results of three shots a few weeks apart and Salk just had to get off his behind and make a speech about how that was the wrong way to do it. He just had to get into the picture. He couldn't keep still and let Tommy have his day. The dosage schedule didn't have to be changed on that day, damn it." Before the day ended, the gulf between Salk and his colleagues was wide and fixed.

On February 22, 1955, about two months before the meeting in Ann Arbor, Jonas Salk appeared on the Edward R. Murrow program, *See It Now.* He responded to a question about his vaccine: "I'd like to say, Mr. Murrow, that this is not the Salk vaccine. This is the polio vaccine. It's come about as a result of contributions made one upon the other not only by men working the field of polio but by others working in related fields. . . . It should be obvious that there was an enormous heritage into which I was born, so to speak, and it's just chance that I happen to be here at this particular time when there was available and at my disposal the great experience of all the investigators who plodded along for a number of years." At the beginning of his speech in Ann Arbor, Salk thanked the staff at the Watson Home and their patients, Basil O'Connor and members of the National Foundation, administrators and trustees of the University of Pittsburgh, and members of his laboratory: "This opportunity would have no meaning if it were not for the devotion with which each of the many of the group that comprises our laboratory contributed and shared in that which needed to be done." Salk was humble and appreciative, but many of his colleagues saw him as a man who actively and brazenly sought a stardom that was beneath that of a real scientist, and they hated him for it.

On April 13, 1955, the day after the announcement in Ann Arbor, the *New York Times* ran the headline "Salk Polio Vaccine Proves Success." The related article stated: "The formal verdict on the Salk vaccine was disclosed . . . amid fanfare and drama far more typical of a Hollywood premiere than a medical meeting." From that day forward, Jonas Salk would be blamed for the fanfare, blamed for the Hollywood atmosphere, blamed for pandering to the media, blamed for putting his name on a vaccine that was at best a temporary solution to the problem of polio, and blamed by many for the tragedy that would soon follow. "I was not unscathed by Ann Arbor," said Salk.

How Does It Feel to Be
a Killer of Children?

4

It's a great day. It's a wonderful day for the whole world. It's a history making day.
—Oveta Culp Hobby, secretary of the Department of Health, Education, and Welfare, moments after signing the licenses for distribution and sale of polio vaccine, April 12, 1955

THE LABORATORY OF BIOLOGICS CONTROL, THE tiny federal agency within the National Institutes of Health responsible for licensing vaccines, was born of a strange event that occurred in the early 1900s. In 1901 a diphtheria epidemic swept across St. Louis, Missouri. Diphtheria was caused by a poison (toxin) released by the bacterium *Corynebacterium diphtheriae*. Diphtheria toxin caused a thick, gray coating on the back of the throat that made it difficult for children to swallow and breathe. The toxin also traveled to the heart, causing heart failure, and to the nervous system, causing paralysis. Sometimes the swelling in the throat was so severe that children died from suffocation. In the early 1900s, diphtheria was one of the most common killers of teenagers in America—as many as two hundred thousand people were infected and fifteen thousand killed by diphtheria every year.

Children were protected against diphtheria by inoculation with "diphtheria antitoxin"—a preparation made by injecting horses with diphtheria toxin and collecting their serum. In the late 1800s and early 1900s many companies and public health agencies made diphtheria antitoxin. In October 1901, during the diphtheria outbreak in St. Louis, five-year-old Veronica Neill received a shot of diphtheria antitoxin. Soon she developed painful spasms of her face and throat, and on October 26 she died—from tetanus.

Tetanus was much less common than diphtheria and was caused by a different bacterium (*Clostridium tetani*). Tetanus bacteria live in the soil and usually enter the body when it is pierced by a rusty nail or piece of glass. But Veronica hadn't cut herself, and she wasn't the only child in St. Louis who died suddenly and unexpectedly from tetanus. Thirteen children died from tetanus that fall, and all had received diphtheria antitoxin from the same batch, made by the city's health department. Veronica's doctor called the health department, and the antitoxin was quickly recalled. An investigation found that one of the horses used to make the diphtheria antitoxin—a milk wagon horse named Jim—had contracted tetanus. As a consequence, deadly tetanus toxin was mistakenly injected into children. A similar incident occurred in the fall of 1901 in Camden, New Jersey, when nine children died from tetanus after receiving a smallpox vaccine contaminated with tetanus bacteria.

In response to these tragedies, on July 2, 1902, Congress enacted and then President Theodore Roosevelt signed into law the Biologics Control Act. The federal government now had the authority to regulate the shipment of "any virus, therapeutic serum, toxin, antitoxin, or analogous product applicable to the prevention and cure of diseases of man."

In 1955 the Laboratory of Biologics Control had an annual budget of $327,000 (about one-twentieth of what it cost to perform the trial of the vaccine it would soon regulate). The staff at the laboratory consisted of forty-five people, ten of whom were either doctors or scientists. Not one member of the laboratory in the spring of 1955 had ever studied polio virus or published a single article on the disease. These ten professionals were responsible for testing 200 separate products and supervising more than 150 establishments.

Although the Laboratory of Biologics Control had granted more than one thousand licenses, the polio license was unique. Never had the testing of a product been so widely known or its license so greatly anticipated. The agency was expected to do things quickly, in the glare of publicity, and under constant pressure from the National Foundation and politicians. "They didn't know how to handle it and they didn't have the expertise to handle it," one former employee recalled.

Prior to 1955, the research, development, and testing of the polio vaccine had been the sole responsibility of the National Foundation. Now the vaccine was in the hands of the Laboratory of Biologics Control. Thomas Rivers and Basil O'Connor decided that after the polio vaccine was licensed, their job was done. But Rivers and O'Connor were apprehensive about passing the baton to the federal government; they felt that no one in the public health service knew anything about polio.

Rivers and O'Connor had reason for concern. There were several critical differences between vaccine made for the field trial (supervised by the National Foundation) and vaccine that was later sold to the public (supervised by the Laboratory of Biologics Control). First, the National Foundation hired companies to make a product according to specifications in the Salk protocol, a document that was fifty-five pages long. The Laboratory of Biologics Control asked manufacturers to comply with a document entitled "Minimum requirements," which was five pages long. By law, companies had to comply with the government document only.

Second, the National Foundation required that each company make at least eleven consecutive lots of vaccine that was free of live virus. The Laboratory of Biologics Control required a "method which [was] consistently effective and reliable in inactivating a series of lots." "Consistently" and "series" were never defined.

Third, the Salk protocol devoted five and one-half pages to the concept and technique of virus inactivation, stressing that inactivation "should be done in such a way that at least *four reliable points* are available for constructing a line that will indicate the rate at which virus infectivity is being destroyed." The time needed to establish a margin of safety was "calculated by tripling the time at which there remain[ed] but one infectious [particle]." In place of these five and one-half pages, the Laboratory of Biologics Control used five sentences. Details on the number of samples to be tested and how long to treat with formaldehyde were never given.

Fourth, the National Foundation required that virus be inactivated with formaldehyde in a "final concentration of 1 to 4000." The Laboratory of Biologics Control used the phrase "*if* formaldehyde is used for inactivation." The government used the word "if" to accommodate

Parke-Davis's interest in using ultraviolet light to inactivate virus. Neither the safety nor the effectiveness of polio vaccine prepared with ultraviolet light had ever been tested in people.

But there was an even bigger flaw in how the government supervised the pharmaceutical companies: manufacturers were not legally required to inform the government about batches of vaccine that failed safety tests. If a batch of polio vaccine contained live polio virus, the company simply didn't submit that lot for approval, and the federal government never knew about its existence. The Laboratory of Biologics Control defended its policy, claiming that manufacturers had "a perfect right to make a batch [that] on the final tests for safety, purity, and potency failed" as long as that lot was never sold to the public.

Immediately after Thomas Francis announced the results of the field trial, at 2:45 P.M. on the afternoon of April 12, 1955, William Workman, the director of the Laboratory of Biologics Control, gathered fifteen people in a hotel room in Ann Arbor. This was the licensing advisory committee, and its task was to determine whether licenses to make polio vaccine should be granted to Eli Lilly, Parke-Davis, Pitman-Moore, Wyeth, and Cutter. Everyone in the room was either a polio expert or a representative of the federal government. Each member of the committee was given a copy of the Francis report of the field trial (113 pages long) and protocols that detailed how each of forty lots of vaccine had been manufactured (each protocol was about 50 pages long). Most members of this group were looking, for the first time, at approximately 2,000 pages of information.

Despite the massive amount of work before them, the advisory committee was pressured to make a decision quickly. Oveta Culp Hobby, the secretary of Health, Education, and Welfare, had arranged a press conference later that day, when she would officially sign the licenses. Hobby was a veteran of public service. She had been the executive vice president of the *Houston Post;* the director of the Women's Army Corps (WACs) during World War II, where she had won the Distinguished Service Medal; and the chairman of the Federal Security Agency. Tough, pragmatic, and resourceful, Hobby was a successful and powerful woman—she expected her demand for a rapid licensing process to be met.

In an uncomfortably small, smoke-filled hotel room in Ann Arbor, Workman's advisory committee sat around a large table to review manufacturers' protocols. Howard Shaughnessy, the director of the laboratory at the Illinois State Health Department, attended the licensing meeting: "As I recall, the Committee was unable to get together until something about 2:45. We were asked to come to a decision very quickly. Mrs. Hobby was waiting on the other end of the line for an answer from us. They wanted us to give the answer by 4:00 o'clock and the Committee demurred that this was certainly pushing it too much, so that we agreed to see if we could come to a decision by 5:00 o'clock of that day. There was discussion, general discussion, of the report that Dr. Francis had given; but we were not in a position to discuss it very intensively because we had not seen the report prior to this morning." After two and one-half hours of discussion, the group unanimously recommended licensure for all five companies. (Today it takes at least one year to license a vaccine, and supportive documents are about sixty thousand pages long.)

Unfortunately the licensing committee never saw one important piece of information. Bernice Eddy, the person at the Laboratory of Biologics Control directly responsible for polio vaccine, had recently told her boss, William Workman, of a disturbing finding. Eddy had accepted the challenge of determining whether commercial lots of polio vaccine contained live polio virus. Although only Parke-Davis and Eli Lilly had made vaccine for the field trial, Pitman-Moore, Wyeth, and Cutter had submitted samples of their vaccines to the laboratory months before licenses were granted. "This was a product that had never been made before and they were going to use it right away," said Eddy. "We had eighteen monkeys. We inoculated these eighteen monkeys with each vaccine that came in." Eddy used a dental drill to make a small hole in the skulls of twelve anesthetized monkeys and injected polio vaccine into their brains. The other six monkeys received polio vaccine by injection into their muscles.

Eddy found that three of the six lots of vaccine submitted by Cutter Laboratories paralyzed monkeys. She later quizzed a colleague, "What do you think is wrong with these monkeys?" "They were given polio," the researcher speculated. "No," Eddy replied, "they were given the polio vaccine." Eddy removed the spinal cords from the monkeys and, to her horror, found live polio virus. She reported these results to William Workman, but Workman never told the licensing committee what Bernice Eddy had found. Although Cutter Laboratories didn't sell these contaminated lots of vaccine to the public, Eddy's finding of live polio virus signaled a critical flaw in Cutter's manufacturing process. "There's going to be a disaster. I know it," she said to a friend.

At 5:15 P.M., one hour after her scheduled press conference and long after her opportunity to share the spotlight with Thomas Francis and Jonas Salk had passed, Oveta Culp Hobby signed the licenses granting permission for five pharmaceutical companies to distribute polio vaccine. That evening, health clinics across the country received cardboard boxes marked "POLIO VACCINE: RUSH."

The day that Oveta Culp Hobby signed the license permitting Cutter Laboratories to sell its vaccine, Julius Youngner boarded a plane to San Francisco to attend a scientific meeting. Youngner, like all members of Salk's laboratory, was saddened by Salk's failure to mention his name during the announcement in Ann Arbor. "We all took it pretty hard," said Youngner; "some cried."

While unpacking at his hotel, Youngner received a telephone call from Ralph Houlihan, associate director of research for Cutter Laboratories.

Houlihan: Do you ever have difficulty getting complete inactivation?

Youngner: What do you mean?

Houlihan: When live virus is supposed to be gone, we still find it for days and days.

Youngner: I can't address your problem without first seeing exactly what you're doing.

Houlihan sent a private car to San Francisco to bring Youngner to Berkeley, the site of Cutter's home office and manufacturing plant. When he arrived, Youngner noticed that the scientists at Cutter were tense and secretive: "They were edgy, very edgy."

Youngner first visited the site where Cutter made polio vaccine. He found an unimpressive single-story structure made of hollow tile, with

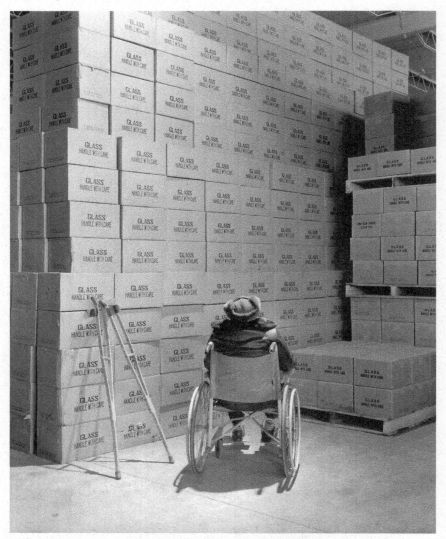

Polio vaccine in crates ready to be shipped across the country; January 11, 1955 (courtesy of the March of Dimes Birth Defects Foundation).

concrete slab floors, painted plaster walls and ceilings, and a stucco exterior. After a tour of the building and a review of the manufacturing records, Julius Youngner was shaken. Cutter was growing live polio virus in the same room in which it stored killed vaccine; its inactivation curves didn't follow the straight line that Youngner had observed in Salk's laboratory; its notebooks were sloppy, its facilities were cramped, and its protocols were illegible or inaccurate. "They looked like they didn't know what the hell they were doing," he said.

In mid-April 1955 Julius Youngner was probably the only person outside of Cutter Laboratories who knew exactly how much trouble Cutter was having inactivating polio virus. When he returned to Pittsburgh, Youngner told Salk about his visit to Cutter and volunteered to write letters to William Workman at the Laboratory of Biologics Control and to Basil O'Connor at the National Foundation, urging the government to withdraw Cutter's vaccine. Salk offered to write the letters himself. But letters were never written. For fifty years Julius Youngner has carried the burden of his inaction. "There is not a day that goes by when I don't feel personally responsible for what happened," said Youngner, gazing at a snow-covered street outside his Pittsburgh home. "I could have done something, but I didn't. I was too trusting, too naïve. I blamed Jonas, but I should only blame myself. I didn't follow up on my request. My relationship with Salk was never the same again. I saw him a few years ago and reminded him of what happened the day I returned from Cutter. He was passive—said nothing, as if he had blanked it out." Other than Salk, Youngner never told anyone else what he saw at Cutter Laboratories.

On April 12 and 13, 1955, the Laboratory of Biologics Control approved thirteen lots of polio vaccine for distribution and sale: six were from Cutter Laboratories, two from Eli Lilly, three from Parke-Davis, and two from Pitman-Moore. Between April 19 and April 21 Cutter released three more lots of vaccine. During the next two weeks, five companies, including Wyeth Laboratories, distributed forty lots of vaccine containing about 5 million doses.

On April 25 Harold Graning, regional medical director for the Public Health Service in Chicago, telephoned William Workman. Thirteen days had passed since children had received their first injections of polio vaccine. Graning told Workman about a one-year-old infant whose legs were completely paralyzed eight days after receiving polio vaccine. The next day at twelve noon, Robert Dyar, a state epidemiologist for the California Health Department, called Workman about two seven-year-old boys from San Diego who were paralyzed in their left arms seven days after receiving polio vaccine. At 2 P.M. Dyar

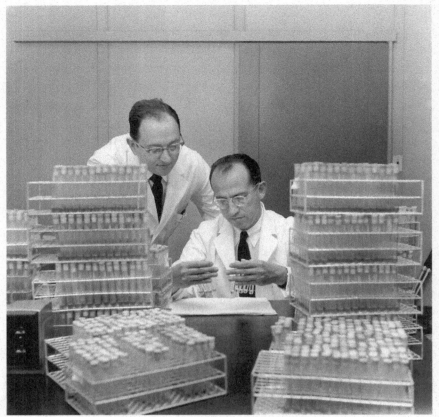

Julius Youngner (left) confers with Jonas Salk; October 1954 (courtesy of the March of Dimes Birth Defects Foundation).

called Workman about a fifteen-month-old boy from Ventura County who was paralyzed in his left arm nine days after receiving vaccine. At 4 P.M. Dyar called Workman again about a twenty-month-old from Napa and a four-year-old from Oakland, both of whom were paralyzed in the left arm after receiving vaccine. Although five companies had made and distributed polio vaccine by April 26, all six paralyzed children had received vaccine made by only one company—Cutter Laboratories.

Twenty years had passed since John Kolmer had injected children with live polio virus and watched as his vaccine caused paralysis and death. During those twenty years, researchers believed that they had learned how to inactivate polio virus and that they had developed sophisticated methods to detect live polio virus in a vaccine. In 1954 they had tested the vaccine in more than four hundred thousand children. Despite the confidence gained by years of experience in refining and perfecting a polio vaccine, William Workman, the man directly responsible for allowing companies to make and sell the vaccine, was reliving the horror of polio's past.

At 6 P.M. on April 26 Workman called his boss, Victor Haas, and Haas in turn called his boss, James Shannon. Shannon and Haas decided to hold an emergency meeting that night that included Workman; David Price, the assistant surgeon general; Alexander Langmuir, chief epidemiologist at the Communicable Disease Center in Atlanta (now the Centers for Disease Control and Prevention); Roderick Murray, the assistant director of the Laboratory of Biologics Control; and Karl Habel, an experienced virologist who worked at the National Institutes of Health. The group met to determine whether Cutter's vaccine had caused paralysis. Because children received only one dose of Salk's vaccine, because Salk's vaccine wasn't 100 percent effective even after three doses, and because polio epidemics still occurred in the United States, it was possible that natural polio had infected the children just before they had received Cutter's vaccine.

First, the group reviewed protocols of specific lots of vaccine implicated in the six cases. What they did not know was that Cutter had sent them only protocols of vaccine lots that had passed safety tests (and had been sold to the public); they didn't know that one-third of Cutter's vaccine had failed the safety tests (and had been incinerated or retreated with formaldehyde). One participant later recalled, "We checked the manufacturing protocols that Cutter had submitted on its batches of vaccine and we saw nothing wrong. We did not find out until some days later that Cutter had been sending us its records only on vaccine that passed the safety tests. But we did not know this on the 26th. We had to play safe, but we didn't want to undermine the immunization program. It was a terribly tense situation."

Next, the group called several representatives of the California Health Department to get more information. Alexander Langmuir found that the cases were alarmingly similar: "When we began to fill in the gaps I became as convinced as anyone could be at this stage that the cases were attributable to a common source, the Cutter vaccine. Each of the children had fallen ill a few days after inoculation. In each case, the first paralysis had occurred at the site of inoculation. No comparable outbreaks of polio seemed to be taking place among unvaccinated children in the same communities."

Finally, the group considered the options. Langmuir felt strongly that all Cutter vaccine should be recalled: "I believed that our one small hope of avoiding catastrophe was to get the Cutter vaccine off the market at once. Bill Workman agreed. But the others voted to wait, figuring that it all might turn out to be a false alarm and that drastic action would be a mistake until we were more certain what was going on."

After seven hours of discussion, the group couldn't agree on a plan. In the early morning hours of April 27 David Price called his boss, Leonard A. Scheele, and told him of the impasse. As the Surgeon General of the United States, Scheele would make the final decision. Figuring that vaccinations would not begin in California until 11:30 A.M. Eastern Standard Time, Scheele decided to delay his decision and asked for a conference of polio experts for early that morning.

Victor Haas arranged a telephone conference for 8 A.M. on April 27, 1955, forty hours after the first report of paralysis following Cutter's vaccine. Haas would direct a meeting that included David Price (assistant surgeon general), Thomas Francis (director of the field trial), Joe Smadel (scientific director at the Walter Reed Army Medical Center), Howard Shaughnessy (director of the laboratory at the Illinois State Health Department), and William McDowall Hammon (professor of epidemiology at the University of Pittsburgh School of Public Health). All were experienced polio researchers. A transcript of this telephone conference reveals that these six men knew there was a problem but didn't know what to do about it.

> Haas: We are calling you at the request of the Surgeon General because of some events that have taken place in the last two days in relation to polio vaccine. There have been several cases of polio reported.

William Workman then described the six cases of polio reported from Chicago and California and the manufacturing protocols submitted by Cutter.

Workman: [The protocols] have been reviewed carefully and were reviewed prior to release of vaccine, and so far as I can tell, the manufacturer's tests have been entirely in accord with the [government] requirements.

Haas: The question we are concerned with, and the question the Surgeon General wants to get opinions on, is what we should do. We could ask the manufacturer to withdraw all vaccine or wait and see what happens, but if we do that— there will be vaccine given today in California. At 3 o'clock this morning, [the California Health Department] said they would be willing to do whatever we recommend.

Haas was asked how much Cutter vaccine had been distributed and how much had been used.

Haas: They have shipped out 165,000 doses. . . . [The] best estimate, which is only a guess, is that perhaps half of those have actually been injected.

Cutter executives, as it turned out, had grossly underestimated how many children had actually been inoculated with their vaccine.

Hammon: I think one ought to be very cautious about having any more Cutter material injected until further data are available.

Smadel: I don't see how you can pick out Cutter and stop all injections; if you are going that far you have to stop the whole business.

Workman: We have no information on anything at all on this so far as the other manufacturers are concerned. I, personally, would like to face the situation with each manufacturer, if and when it develops.

Hammon: I don't think that we have any right to penalize the other manufacturers at this time. I think everything should be directed toward [Cutter].

Haas: We have two opinions here, if I understand it correctly. One is to terminate all of Cutter's vaccine immediately and the other is to pinpoint this action on two or at the most four lots. Is that right?

Francis: Without knowing what has been used anywhere else, we are still talking blind. You are asking questions on which you do not have enough data to permit anything further than a guess.

Workman: On the basis of the [protocols], I have no reason whatever to suspect one lot any more than another of Cutter's product.

Smadel: Well, that puts you on the spot.

Haas: Would anyone raise serious objections if the Surgeon General decided, on the basis of what we can determine now, to discontinue all use of Cutter material immediately?

Smadel: I think that is fairly stringent.

Hammon: I would be in favor of going a little further than Dr. Smadel has suggested. . . . I think one ought to be very cautious about having any more Cutter material injected until further data are available.

Haas: How would you feel, for the sake of the record, if the Surgeon General did nothing at all?

Smadel: I think he had better do something.

The group was unable to form a clear, single plan. Victor Haas later recalled the meeting: "All agreed the Surgeon General should take some action, but they couldn't agree on what it should be. They were not even of one mind on whether he should stop the use of Cutter vaccine. They preferred not to halt the whole program, but they said they would go along with whatever the Surgeon General decided to do."

Two groups of doctors and scientists had weighed their options; neither was able to make a decision. Now it was up to the Surgeon General of the United States, Leonard A. Scheele. The forty-seven-year-old Scheele, a "tall solid relaxed man with a youthful, unlined face" was a son of the Midwest. Born in Fort Wayne, Indiana, Scheele graduated from the University of Michigan and received his medical degree from the Detroit College of Medicine and Surgery (now Wayne State University School of Medicine). From the beginning of his professional career, Scheele was interested in public health. After internship, he began a series of rotations in quarantine stations in San Francisco, San Pedro, and Honolulu. Days after the attack on Pearl Harbor, Scheele reported to the medical department of the army and later served in Italy, Germany, and Africa. In 1948 he was appointed surgeon general. Three years later, on April 24, 1951, Leonard Scheele issued an unqualified recommendation for the fluoridation of public drinking water—a recommendation that was at the time very controversial.

On the morning of April 27, 1955, Scheele had several options. He

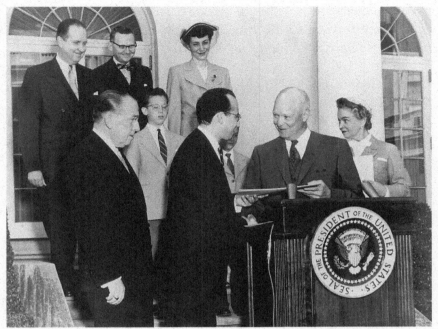

President Dwight David Eisenhower presents the U.S. Medal of Merit to
Jonas Salk on April 23, 1955, in a ceremony at the White House Rose Gar-
den. The presentation, which occurred two days before the first child was
paralyzed by polio vaccine, was observed by Oveta Culp Hobby (front
right), Basil O'Connor (front left), Surgeon General Leonard Scheele (back
left), and Donna Salk (back right). Salk's children Peter (center) and Darrell
(partially obscured) were also present (courtesy of the March of Dimes
Birth Defects Foundation).

could do nothing—and risk more cases of paralysis caused by Cutter's
vaccine. He could recall only the lots of Cutter's vaccine associated
with the six reported cases—and risk paralysis caused by other lots of
Cutter's vaccine. He could recall all lots of Cutter's vaccine—and risk
paralysis caused by vaccine made by other companies. Or he could
recall all polio vaccines—and risk sacrificing children to an epidemic of
polio that was poised to sweep across the country in a few months.

Scheele had one other problem. He couldn't force Cutter Laboratories to recall its vaccine. The Biologics Control Act gave the federal
government the authority to license a vaccine but not the authority to

stop a company from selling a vaccine that was already licensed. If Scheele decided that Cutter's vaccine should be withdrawn, the company would have to withdraw it voluntarily.

Cutter Laboratories was founded by Edward Ahern ("E. A.") Cutter. The son and grandson of physicians and community leaders, E. A. Cutter was born and raised in Sutton, Quebec, a small village south of Montreal. When he was eighteen years old, E. A. moved to Traver, California, in the San Joaquin Valley, to become an apprentice pharmacist. In the late 1800s, Traver was a town alive with commerce and energy, but when a rail line that would later become the Santa Fe Railroad was built on the east side of the valley, Traver deteriorated badly. So E. A. moved to San Jacinto, California, where he bought a small drugstore in the center of town. At the back of the store, in a room approximately eight feet by eight feet, he set up a laboratory. The laboratory served local doctors by performing tests on blood and urine.

In 1897, at age twenty-seven, E. A. Cutter moved from San Jacinto to Fresno, California, married, and bought another drugstore—the first in town to have an ice cream parlor. Again E. A. set up a diagnostic laboratory in the back and called it Cutter Analytic Laboratory. The laboratory analyzed urine (to determine the presence of bacteria), blood (to determine the number of white and red blood cells), and sputum (to determine whether patients were infected with diphtheria or tuberculosis). Guinea pigs, used to test for bacterial infections, were kept in a bathtub in the back of the store.

In 1903 Cutter Analytic Laboratory moved from Fresno to Berkeley and became Cutter Laboratories. One of the first pharmaceutical companies in the United States, Cutter's flagship product was black-leg vaccine. Blackleg was a disease of cattle caused by a bacterium (*Clostridium chauvei*). Calves with blackleg developed high fever, loss of appetite, lameness, and swelling of the muscles. As the disease progressed, the muscles liquefied, became swollen and black, and produced a crackling sound when pressed by hand because of the gas produced by the growing bacteria (also known as gas gangrene). Because blackleg was an important cause of disease and death in California cattle, cattlemen wanted to find a way to prevent it.

To make blackleg vaccine, E. A. Cutter—later helped by his three sons, Robert, Ted, and Fred—removed the bacteria and its poisons, called toxins, from the affected muscles and inactivated them with a chemical. Ted Cutter remembered helping his father make blackleg vaccine: "I can remember very well the smelly job I had, which was the production of blackleg [toxin]. They brought the calf down by injecting him with virulent blackleg [bacteria]. Then, after he died, they took the muscle tissue and expressed all the juice . . . and collected it into jars and such. And the odor just permeated not only your clothes, but your skin and everything." Marketed under the name "Blacklegol Bacterin," blackleg vaccine sold for ten cents a dose.

Cutter Laboratories also made other veterinary vaccines: hog cholera vaccine, to prevent a severe and often fatal infection of pigs; horse encephalomyelitis vaccine, to prevent a debilitating nervous system disease of horses; and anthrax vaccine, to prevent a fatal respiratory disease of cattle.

Cutter also made vaccines for people. The first two human vaccines it made were for smallpox and rabies. As a teenager, Robert Cutter, who would later run Cutter Laboratories, helped make smallpox vaccine: "[Calves] were put on a table with their feet upright and strapped to four rising wooden bars," Cutter recalled. "Their belly was shaved and then [abraded] by light scratches. . . . The vaccine was placed on the calf's belly, and then the calf was held for . . . a few days, sacrificed— and the vaccine was harvested by means of curettes or spoons with sharp edges. I know all about that because that was later one of my jobs." The smallpox vaccine was first sold by Cutter in 1904.

Cutter Laboratories is best known today for the insect repellent that bears its name, but between 1910 and 1955 it introduced many innovative and successful medical products. In response to a need to prevent tetanus during World War I, Cutter was the first company to make tetanus antitoxin in the United States; it also made antitoxins against diphtheria and streptococcus. Antitoxins were made using horses that were kept in a small stable nearby. Cutter was among the first companies to make vaccines against diphtheria, tetanus, and pertussis (whooping cough), and it was the first company in the world to combine these three vaccines into a single shot. The combined vaccine (also known as DTP) was used for decades in the United States.

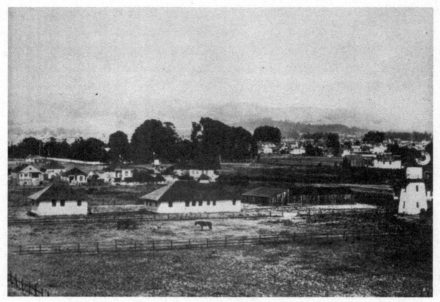

Cutter Laboratories, 1903. Horses used to make antitoxins are in the fore-
ground (courtesy of the Bayer Corporation).

Cutter was the first company in the United States to enhance immune responses to vaccines by adding a chemical called aluminum
hydroxide. (Aluminum hydroxide and other aluminum salts are used
in many human vaccines today.)

Cutter was among the first companies to make blood products
(such as plasma) and to mass produce penicillin during World War II,
and it was the only company to continue to make blood products after
the war ended.

Cutter revolutionized the field of intravenous solutions (fluids
given by vein). Before Cutter's entrance into the field, solutions containing sugars and minerals could be given only under the skin or into
the muscle; they couldn't be given intravenously because the bottles,
flasks, and plastics used to administer them often contained pyrogens,
substances that caused high fever and occasionally fatal reactions. Cutter Laboratories developed nonpyrogenic flasks and tubing (produced
under the trade name Saftiflask), and for the first time fluids that re-
stored lost water and minerals could be given intravenously. Intravenous solutions were so popular that they created markets in the East
and Midwest for Cutter's other products.

Cutter was also one of the first companies to have a medical product recalled. In April 1948 it sent more than 2,900 bottles of a solution containing glucose (sugar) in normal saline (salt water) to hospitals in Florida, Kentucky, Mississippi, Alabama, and Georgia. The solutions were found to be cloudy—probably because they were contaminated with bacteria or fungi—and several people died following their use. The Food and Drug Administration immediately issued a severe warning and asked for the withdrawal of all unused bottles. Charged with "misbranding and adulteration," Cutter appeared in a California court the following year, pleaded no contest, and paid a fine of $600.

By April 1955 Cutter Laboratories was run by E. A. Cutter's eldest son, Robert. A member of the Sierra Club, the National Rifle Association, and the Audubon Society, Robert Cutter was an outdoorsman whose passion led him to try to breed the first aromatic camellia. After graduating from Yale Medical School in 1923, Robert practiced medicine for three years in Oakland, California, before joining Cutter Laboratories as assistant medical director; within four years he was running the company. A relentlessly upbeat, positive man in excellent physical condition, Robert Cutter "didn't walk, he sprung and bounced." Later Ted Cutter, who served as executive vice-president, and Fred Cutter, who served as vice president and secretary, joined Robert in running Cutter Laboratories.

In 1955 Cutter was a modest pharmaceutical company with $11.5 million in annual sales. Despite its small size relative to companies such as Parke-Davis and Eli Lilly, the National Foundation approached Cutter Laboratories because, as Robert Cutter recalled, "we were pioneers, really, in tissue vaccines through our work in the veterinary field." When the National Foundation asked it to make Salk's polio vaccine, Cutter decided to deemphasize its blood products business. "We saw this polio vaccine as a great opportunity for us to increase our sales and our earnings," recalled Henry Lange, Cutter's chief financial officer.

To head its polio vaccine program, Robert Cutter picked Walter Ward. An "extremely thin individual" who looked like an "ascetic Japanese elder or a Tibetan monk," Ward received both a PhD and an MD from the University of Chicago and completed residency training in medicine at the University of Southern California. Hired in 1946,

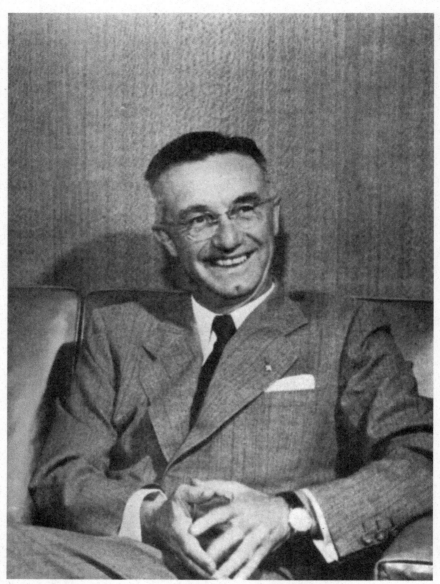
Robert K. Cutter, 1954 (courtesy of the Bayer Corporation).

Ward was by 1955 the director of medical research for all human products. Those who worked for him and with him described Ward as distant, haughty, secretive, and pedantic.

Ward oversaw all aspects of the polio manufacturing process: he reviewed all protocols detailing how polio virus was grown; he reviewed all graphs showing how polio virus was inactivated; and he reviewed all vaccine safety tests. He was responsible for signing off on every lot of vaccine and for submitting protocols for approval to the Laboratory of Biologics Control. In the end, Walter Ward was the only person at Cutter Laboratories who knew exactly what was happening with the polio vaccine at every stage of processing, development, and testing.

Throughout 1954 and early 1955 five pharmaceutical companies competed to be the first on the market with a polio vaccine. Cutter Laboratories won the contest. It made six of the first thirteen lots approved by the Laboratory of Biologics Control. As a reward to its staff members for their hard work, in mid-April 1955 Cutter executives cleared the cafeteria, brought in nurses, and gave the vaccine to the children of 450 employees.

Leonard Scheele decided to ask Cutter Laboratories to recall all of its vaccine, not just the lots that were associated with paralysis. On Wednesday, April 27, 1955, at 10:00 A.M., William Workman of the Laboratory of Biologics Control sent a telegram to Walter Ward of Cutter Laboratories:

> YOU ARE REQUESTED TO DISCONTINUE DISTRIBUTION OF POLIOMYELITIS VAC-
> CINE UNTIL FURTHER NOTICE AND TO WITHDRAW ALL ISSUED UNUSED PACKAGES
> FROM THE MARKET. KINDLY NOTIFY ALL CONSIGNEES OF POLIOMYELITIS VACCINE
> ACCORDINGLY.
>
> PLEASE DELIVER AT ONCE!

Cutter complied. Thirty-eight minutes later, it sent a telegram to all health departments and drug stores that had received its vaccine:

> URGENT. NO FURTHER INJECTIONS OF CUTTER POLIO VACCINE ARE TO BE MADE.
> IMMEDIATELY ADVISE YOUR PHYSICIANS. PLEASE RETURN UNUSED SUPPLIES OF
> POLIOMYELITIS VACCINE.

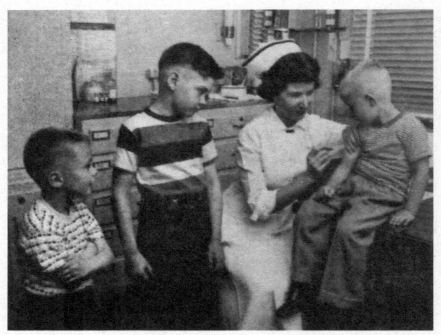

Richard Taylor, son of Cutter employee and polio researcher Ken Taylor, is vaccinated with Cutter vaccine in April 1955. Brothers Paul and Stanley wait their turn (courtesy of the Bayer Corporation).

After Cutter Laboratories sent out its telegram, Robert Cutter issued a press release: "Symptoms diagnosed as polio have been reported as occurring in several children who have received Cutter Poliomyelitis Vaccine. It is not known whether there is any relationship to the injection. However, in view of the serious possibilities, the only proper and safe course is to immediately stop any further use." But Robert Cutter still hoped that his vaccine was not to blame. "There have been symptoms reported in seven cases out of over three-quarters of a million doses issued by Cutter," he said. "One of these has, however, already been ruled out."

Although all six paralyzed children had received vaccine made by Cutter and despite the fact that five of the six were paralyzed in the arm that was inoculated, Leonard Scheele issued his own statement: "I want first and foremost to assure the parents of children who have received an injection of polio vaccine this spring that in the very best judgment of the Public Health Service, they have no cause for alarm." But there was cause for alarm. The same day that Scheele issued his statement, two more children were reported paralyzed; both were from Idaho, and both had been inoculated with Cutter's vaccine. One child was paralyzed in the left arm, and the other died nine days after the injection.

By April 29, within twenty-four hours of the recall, the number of victims of Cutter's vaccine had reached eleven—all in the West and Midwest. Scheele continued to try to calm public fears, saying that the withdrawal of Cutter's vaccine "does not imply that there is any correlation between the vaccine and the occurrence of polio." Robert Cutter also continued to express hope that his vaccine was not at fault. "Retesting has already begun," said Cutter. "There is only one thing to do—run down every possible clue. We cannot possibly let any of the vaccine out until we are sure . . . no single lot of the vaccine has been implicated and we hope that no lot, nor the vaccine, is implicated."

By April 30, within forty-eight hours of the recall, Cutter's vaccine had paralyzed or killed twenty-five children: fourteen in California, seven in Idaho, two in Washington, one in Illinois, and one in Colorado.

At 4:00 P.M. on April 27, within hours of hearing about the withdrawal of Cutter's vaccine, Jonas Salk issued a calm, measured statement to the press: "I have just learned of the decision by the Public Health Service. It is difficult to say whether or not the association between vaccination and the reported cases is one of cause and effect or one of coincidence. . . . It would seem that what is being done is reasonable, namely that a thorough investigation of the reported cases is being made." Privately Salk was heartbroken. Donna Salk remembered that "[Jonas] was concerned; he was worried; he was anxious; he was depressed. But not because he thought there was something wrong with [his process] at all. It was more like, 'How could this happen? How could this be allowed to happen?'" Jonas Salk shared his feelings with a friend who recalled, "He was never optimistic except in terms of what he was doing in his own lab and he was scared shitless about what was happening or could happen in some of these pharmaceutical factories. He thought that some were not paying attention and that others were just slobs. [After the recall] he retreated. He hadn't done anything wrong. Whatever had happened had been the result of a foul-up at Cutter. He felt that there was no real excuse for that kind of fumbling at a time when it was possible to inoculate millions of people—especially children—and fortify them for life. He was terribly upset about this long after the fact."

Some scientists used the incident to attack Salk and his vaccine. Thomas Weller, who had shared the Nobel Prize one year earlier for figuring out how to grow polio virus in cell culture, called Salk's vaccine "one of the biggest scientific farces ever foisted on the public. It was just no damn good."

The National Foundation had distributed vaccine free of charge to all first and second graders. But pharmaceutical companies also sold the vaccine, and many doctors gave the vaccine to teenagers and adults. The New York County Medical Society accused six physicians of violating the unofficial priorities of inoculating children first. Further, several prominent physicians received vaccine from companies as a gesture of good will. Alton Ochsner, a professor of surgery at Tulane Medical School and founder of the Ochsner Clinic in New Orleans, had received samples of Cutter's vaccine. Ochsner, a renowned cancer surgeon, was the first physician to recognize the association between cigarette smoking and lung cancer—a theory he published with student Michael De Bakey in 1939. Ochsner gave Cutter's vaccine to his grandson, Eugene ("Davey") Davis and watched the boy die as a result. John Ochsner, the child's uncle, recalled the tragedy: "He was a beautiful little boy, a doll of a boy, and the love of my father's life. When Davey died my father's heart was broken."

Tom Coleman, a medical writer who had worked with Salk, remembered the panic: "I was on the telephone for more than twenty-four hours. Physicians at that time were limited to immunizing infants. But 90 percent of the calls I received were from physicians who had given the vaccine to their kids, mothers, aunts, and neighbors and were worried about what would happen."

Cutter's employees and executives were humiliated by the recall. Robert Routh worked with Frank Deromedi on vaccine production. Sitting at his kitchen table in a small, one-story brick home in Livermore, California, not far from Cutter Laboratories, Routh remembered the excitement among the employees at the beginning of the

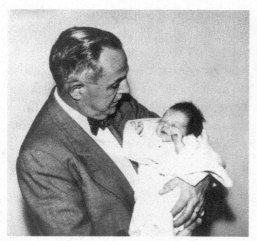 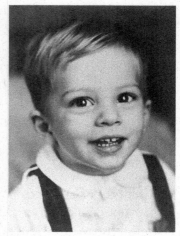

Renowned surgeon Alton Ochsner holds his infant grandson, Eugene ("Davey") Davis (left). The child was inoculated with Cutter vaccine when he was two years old (right) and died as a consequence (photos courtesy of John Ochsner).

polio project: "It was an uplifting challenge. Here's something we can get into. We know how to make vaccines. We'd been making vaccines for years. People worked their tails off on that. But when these first reports came in that people who had gotten the vaccine were coming down with polio, it was 'Oh, my God! How could this be?' No one at the time had the faintest idea what could possibly have gone wrong. We knew that we had followed the manufacturing and testing protocols right down to the gnat's eyelashes." "We panicked," said co-worker Deromedi, who had immunized his sons, Dennis, age eight, and Craig, age five. "After all, our kids had been vaccinated."

Robert Cutter was besieged by the press. In the lobby of Cutter's main building, news reporters and cameramen crowded in on a man who loved the freedom and solace of the outdoors. "All I could say is, 'We don't know,'" recalled Cutter. "They tried to put words in my mouth and did put words in my mouth and a photographer hovered around, taking pictures of me. In one of the magazines, which was the epitome of yellow journalism at the time—I think it was called *Confidential* . . . if I have ever in my life looked like an ogre, I did in that picture. So, the whole thing was to make us look like people who didn't think a thing about killing a child if it meant a dollar to us. It was really terrible."

Other members of the Cutter family were attacked. Robert's son, David, a salesman for Cutter Laboratories at the time of the tragedy, remembered an incident with a member of his family: "My cousin Carol, Ted's daughter, who was a school teacher in Reno at the time, got a few threatening phone calls—anonymous phone calls. I remember her relating one. There was a voice at the other end: 'How does it feel to be a killer of children?' Click."

Cutter's polio vaccine was recalled within forty-eight hours of the first reports of suspected cases. But it was too late; three hundred eighty thousand children had already been inoculated. During the next few months the government sifted through the facts to determine the number of people paralyzed and killed by Cutter's vaccine. This grim accounting would find Cutter Laboratories at the center of one of the worst biological disasters in American history.

A Man-Made Polio Epidemic

I cannot escape a terrible feeling of identification with these people
who got polio.
—Jonas Salk's reaction to the Cutter Incident

ON SUNDAY, APRIL 24, 1955, J. E. WYATT, THE HEALTH
officer in charge of Idaho's southeast district, received a phone call
from a local physician about a girl in Pocatello. "I've just seen a young-
ster who seems to have polio," the doctor said. "Her mother says she
noticed a little stiffness of the neck yesterday and she had fever. Today
her left arm became paralyzed. Her name is Susan Pierce."

Wyatt was aware of the field trial of Salk's vaccine. He knew that
more than four hundred thousand children had received the vaccine
the year before without incident. Reassured by these results, Wyatt
told the physician: "She must have been exposed [to natural polio
virus] before the vaccination, and there wasn't time enough for the
vaccine to protect her. But I'm glad you called. We'll keep a close
watch on things."

Susan's case was baffling. She and her nine-year-old brother, Kenneth, were inoculated with polio vaccine on April 18. Five days later,
she developed fever and neck stiffness. Six days later, her left arm was
paralyzed. Seven days later, she was placed in an iron lung, and nine
days later, she was dead. Kenneth was fine. Her father, Lester Pierce,
"didn't know how she became exposed to the germ" because he didn't
know anyone else who was sick. Her school principal, Lewis Dunn,
said that there were no other cases of polio at Susan's school. And it
was April. Although several hundred cases of polio occurred in Idaho
every year, the first few cases didn't usually appear until June.

Susan was the first of many. On April 26 six-year-old Jimmy Ship-
ley was admitted to the hospital with paralysis of his left arm. On

April 30 Bonnie Gale Pound of Lewiston was admitted to St. Joseph's Hospital with paralysis of her breathing muscles; attempting to save her life, the Idaho Air National Guard flew an iron lung from Boise to Lewiston. Between May 1 and 3 seven-year-old Jimmy Gilbert of Orofino developed paralysis in his left arm, eight-year-old Dorothy Crowley of Alsahka was placed in an iron lung, and Janet Lee Kincaid of Moscow and Danny Eggers of Idaho Falls died from the disease. Every one of these Idaho schoolchildren had received vaccine made by Cutter Laboratories.

Idaho had taken full advantage of the National Foundation's offer to provide vaccine free of charge to all first and second graders. With remarkable efficiency, beginning on April 19, 1955, thirty-two thousand school children—98 percent of Idaho's first and second graders— were immunized with polio vaccine. Every dose was obtained from Cutter Laboratories, and every dose was given before April 28, the day that Cutter Laboratories recalled its vaccine.

The task of determining who was paralyzed and who was killed by Cutter's vaccine fell to Alexander Langmuir, the chief epidemiologist at the Communicable Diseases Center in Atlanta. An engaging, challenging, opinionated man with a "flare for the dramatic," Langmuir was the first to use the term "the Cutter Incident."

Langmuir had to find a way to separate cases of polio caused by Cutter's vaccine from cases of natural polio that coincidentally followed vaccination. The task wouldn't be easy. Three hundred and eighty thousand children had received Cutter's polio vaccine. The National Foundation had provided vaccine for three hundred thousand first and second graders in six western states (California, Idaho, Arizona, Nevada, New Mexico, and Hawaii). Older children, teenagers, and adults in twenty-six states received the remaining eighty thousand doses. Fortunately, five years earlier, Langmuir had created a system that would prove to be invaluable in calculating the impact of Cutter's vaccine.

In December 1950, in the midst of the Cold War, the Federal Civil Defense Administration published two manuals about biological warfare. The manuals warned that agents such as botulism, plague, smallpox, cholera, and anthrax might be sprayed over cities in deadly aerosols or put into supplies of food and water. Langmuir imagined a frightening series of events: "Let us assume that enemy planes succeeded in penetrating our military defenses and that a cloud of infectious aerosol had been laid down upon an unprepared and unsuspecting city. Let us further assume that the concentration of this agent in the cloud was sufficient to produce casualties. . . . What would be the ensuing course of events? Days or weeks later cases of disease would appear. . . . Medical care facilities would be grossly overtaxed. . . . Laboratories would be swamped with specimens . . . [and a] mass exodus from the city might well get started. Confusion would abound and the consequences would be disastrous."

To prevent panic and uncertainty in the face of a biological attack, Langmuir proposed the creation of a new federal emergency response team: "Let us contrast this hypothetical situation with another in which the defense organization was adequately prepared. . . . An alert local laboratory would immediately institute a series of tests designed to identify the specific agent. . . . Through a sound intelligence system, the beginning of the epidemic might well be appreciated hours or even days before it was clearly apparent to any single physician or hospital. . . . The contributions the epidemiologist can make in this defense plan are evident." On April 5, 1951, Alexander Langmuir realized his vision, and the Epidemic Intelligence Service was born.

Langmuir and his team—twenty-two medical officers, seventy-three officials from state and local health departments, nineteen physical therapists, fifteen virus laboratories, and twenty-five laboratory personnel—were prepared to respond to biological attacks by enemies outside of the United States; they never imagined an inadvertent biological attack from a pharmaceutical company inside the country. But on April 28, 1955, Surgeon General Leonard Scheele called on the Epidemic Intelligence Service to investigate the Cutter tragedy. It was the agency's first real assignment. Langmuir and his team gathered information about every case of polio that occurred in 1955; they determined the age, residence, and symptoms of every victim; they determined who had received polio vaccine and who had had contact with someone that had received polio vaccine; they determined who had gotten which specific lots of vaccine; they determined who was shedding polio virus from the intestines and what types of polio virus were being shed; they determined the incidence of polio that had occurred in the spring of each of the preceding five years and compared it with the incidence of polio in the spring of 1955.

Langmuir and his team determined the incidence of paralysis in children who had received vaccine from each of eight production pools made by Cutter Laboratories. They found that for children receiving vaccine from six of the pools the incidence of paralysis was the same as the average incidence of paralysis in children in the spring of the preceding five years. But for children receiving vaccine from two of the production pools (lots 19468 and 19764), the incidence of paralysis was almost ten times greater than expected. Every first and second grader in Idaho had received polio vaccine obtained from Cutter lot 19468.

Langmuir and his team determined that these two lots of Cutter's vaccine had paralyzed fifty-one children and killed five. They also found that the disease caused by Cutter's vaccine was worse than the disease caused by natural polio virus. Children given Cutter's vaccine were more likely to be paralyzed in their arms, more likely to suffer severe and permanent paralysis, more likely to require breathing assistance in iron lungs, and more likely to die than children naturally infected with polio.

Why was the disease caused by Cutter's vaccine more serious and more deadly than natural polio? The answer lies in the virus found in the spinal fluids and intestines of children injected with Cutter's vaccine: Mahoney—the most lethal polio strain. Children injected with Cutter's vaccine had high fever as the virus entered their bloodstreams; nausea and vomiting as the virus entered their intestines; and headache, stiff neck, and paralysis of the breathing muscles as the virus entered their spinal cords. Because natural strains of polio virus were likely to be less damaging than the Mahoney strain and because they weren't directly injected into the muscles of the arm, children infected with Cutter's vaccine were actually worse off than children attacked by natural polio virus.

But the 51 children paralyzed and the 5 killed were only a fraction of those who were harmed by Cutter's vaccine. A study performed in 1957 by an orthopedic surgeon in Idaho, Manley Shaw, revealed exactly how many doses of Cutter's polio vaccine contained live virus. Shaw examined the medical records of 425 schoolchildren from Pocatello, Boise, and Lewiston. He found that about one-third of these children had symptoms of abortive polio: fever, sore throat, headache, vomiting, muscle pain, stiff neck, stiff back, or slight limp; many had persistent muscle weakness up to nine months after receiving vaccine. This meant that at least one out of every three doses of contaminated lots of Cutter vaccine (120,000 doses) contained live polio virus; therefore, it is likely that abortive polio occurred in at least 40,000 children (one-third of 120,000). Further, because abortive polio developed in only about one of every three children infected with natural polio, it is likely that all 120,000 children injected with Cutter's vaccine were injected with live virulent polio virus.

The Cutter tragedy didn't end with those injected with Cutter's vaccine. On May 8, eleven days after the recall of Cutter's vaccine, a twenty-eight-year-old mother visiting Atlanta from Knoxville was hospitalized with polio and put on a ventilator. Because she had never received polio vaccine, investigators assumed that she was another of natural polio's many victims. But one month earlier her two children had received Cutter's vaccine. The next morning a young mother who was a neighbor of Alexander Langmuir's secretary in Atlanta died of polio. Like the Knoxville woman, the neighbor had never received vaccine and, like the Knoxville woman, her baby had received Cutter's vaccine one month earlier. Langmuir, who lived in Atlanta, realized that polio virus was spreading from vaccinated children to others and that the epidemic had traveled to the doorstep of the Communicable Diseases Center. "It was a remarkable and fortuitous coincidence that both of these cases occurred in Atlanta," he recalled.

Langmuir feared the worst: Cutter's vaccine was at the center of a man-made polio epidemic. Langmuir's team found seventy-four unvaccinated family members that were paralyzed—half were parents and half were brothers and sisters of children that had received Cutter's vaccine. One of the family members was a mother who was eight months pregnant; on May 12, she died of polio after contracting the disease from her one-year-old son.

The symptoms of polio in these seventy-four family members were

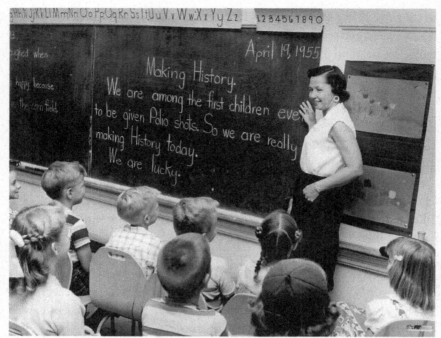

Dorothy Johnson of Boulder City, Nebraska, stands in front of a black-board where she has written, "We are among the first children ever to be given polio shots. So we are really making history today. We are lucky." The statement was written on April 19, 1955—seven days after Cutter Laboratories released its vaccine (courtesy of the March of Dimes Birth Defects Foundation).

different from symptoms in children injected with Cutter's vaccine. They weren't paralyzed in the left arm because they hadn't been injected there. But like the vaccinated children, many family members were severely paralyzed; thirteen required iron lungs and five died from the disease. The high incidence of severe and fatal disease in both vaccinated children and family contacts occurred because they had one thing in common: they were all infected with deadly Mahoney virus.

Spread of the Mahoney virus wasn't limited to family members. On April 16 an infant received an injection of Cutter's vaccine from one of the two tainted production pools. Although the infant never developed symptoms of polio, Mahoney virus was found in her intestines. Three weeks later, her mother developed polio. The mother and infant visited two families who lived nearby. The father in one family and the mother and one child in the second family were paralyzed; the Mahoney strain was isolated from six of eight of these family members. Children in these two families then played with children in a third group of families. Two more children were paralyzed, and eight of nine family members from this third group shed Mahoney virus in their intestines. Many other people who came in contact with infected children were affected; when the outbreak was over, thirty-nine friends and neighbors of children who received Cutter's vaccine were paralyzed.

Given the findings of Manley Shaw in Idaho, it is likely that the Mahoney virus present in Cutter's vaccine infected at least 100,000 family and community contacts. In the end, at least 220,000 people were infected with live polio virus contained in Cutter's vaccine; 70,000 developed muscle weakness, 164 were severely paralyzed, and 10 were killed. Seventy-five percent of Cutter's victims were paralyzed for the rest of their lives. "I wish we'd never heard of the vaccine," Robert Cutter later remarked.

Cutter Laboratories had performed a series of tests to determine whether live virus was present in its vaccine. Before each lot of Cutter's vaccine was given to schoolchildren, Cutter injected it into the brains of twenty-four monkeys, into the muscles of twelve monkeys, and onto monkey kidney cells contained in at least ten separate flasks. The monkeys didn't develop paralysis, and the cells didn't die. But laboratory tests weren't sensitive enough to predict what would happen when the vaccine was injected directly into the arms of hundreds of thousands of children.

On April 27, 1955, within hours of learning about possible problems with Cutter's vaccine, William Workman called Karl Habel and William Tripp into his office, instructing them to go to Cutter Laboratories and find out what happened. That night Habel and Tripp boarded a plane for San Francisco, and the next morning they began their investigation.

Thin and wiry, Karl Habel was a meticulous, thoughtful, and energetic scientist. After graduating from Jefferson Medical College, he completed residency training at Philadelphia General Hospital and the Philadelphia Hospital for Contagious Diseases; he continued his studies at the National Institutes of Health, investigating viruses that damaged the nervous system, such as mumps, rabies, and polio. Later Karl Habel would be one of the first scientists in the world to find unique proteins on the surface of cancer cells. William Tripp received a PhD in chemistry from Purdue, worked on the production of vaccines and antitoxins for the Michigan Department of Health, and in 1950 came to work for William Workman at the Laboratory of Biologics Control.

On the morning of April 28, 1955, Karl Habel and William Tripp arrived at Cutter Laboratories. They found that the building used to make polio vaccine was "in good repair, clean, and generally suitable to the purpose." What surprised Habel and Tripp soon after they arrived was exactly how much trouble Cutter was having. Of twenty-seven production pools of polio vaccine made by Cutter Laboratories, nine contained live polio virus after treatment with formaldehyde. Therefore, only about two-thirds of Cutter's vaccine was potentially usable; the rest was retreated with formaldehyde or placed in an incinerator and burned. Worse, five of the last seven lots of vaccine made by Cutter had contained live virus on safety testing. Apparently Cutter wasn't getting better with experience.

As required by the federal government, Cutter performed two different safety tests: inoculation of vaccine into monkey kidney cells and injection of vaccine into the muscles and brains of monkeys. None of the vaccine sold by Cutter had failed these tests. But Habel found that Cutter's safety tests were worrisomely inconsistent: there was no correlation between the length of time that virus was treated with formaldehyde and the ability of vaccine to pass safety tests; duplicate samples of vaccine contained live virus after inoculation of one flask of cells but not after inoculation of another; individual polio strains (specifically types 1, 2, and 3) passed safety tests, but when pooled together for the final vaccine, they failed; and some lots of vaccine didn't paralyze monkeys inoculated for safety tests but paralyzed monkeys inoculated for potency tests (to see whether vaccine could induce polio antibodies). Habel and Tripp concluded that the safety tests were inadequate and that "small amounts of live virus may be present in the [vaccine] and not be demonstrated by either the tissue culture or monkey tests." They were confident that they could figure out what Cutter was doing wrong.

For the next two weeks, Habel and Tripp worked sixteen hours a day. They transcribed every detail of every lot of Cutter's vaccine. Fifteen secretaries, often working double shifts, traveled from Bethesda to Berkeley to help. After reviewing between six thousand and eight thousand separate records, Habel said: "The records appear complete and adequate [and the inactivation] procedure was being carried out according to what at that time was accepted as routine methods. [There was] nothing different about the procedures at Cutter that I could see."

Habel and Tripp talked to executives Robert Cutter, Fred Cutter, and Ted Cutter, to vaccine production directors Ralph Houlihan and Walter Ward, and to every employee involved in the manufacture of polio vaccine. They found that "Every employee has been completely cooperative and helpful. There have not been any delaying or diverting activities. There has not appeared to be any reluctance to answer any question and we have not noted any conflicting replies, conflicting entries in records, or any evidence of dishonesty or falsification. There has not been any evidence of 'gagging' employees and there has been no incident to discredit any individual. People seemed quite competent. They seemed to know what they were doing and why they were doing it."

Habel and Tripp examined every incubator, refrigerator, sterilizer, ventilation duct, piece of equipment, and laboratory space used in the production of Cutter's vaccine. Again they could not find a single meaningful clue as to what had gone wrong.

Growing desperate, Habel and Tripp investigated the possibility of sabotage. On May 5, 1955, William Tripp sent a letter to Walter Ward that included a list of sixty-seven Cutter employees and asked two questions: "(1) Is there any evidence to indicate that any of the above employees might deliberately subvert the national polio program because of a desire to harm the interests of the United States in contrast to the interests of a foreign country? (2) Have any of the employees been suspected of dishonesty or known to have falsified records in the past?" Five days later Ward answered: "In response to your letter of May 5, 1955, we have reviewed the personnel files of all persons who have access to the polio vaccine. . . . There is no evidence in the files, nor do I have any knowledge that any of the employees might have reason to tamper with the polio vaccine. In this connection, I might point out that all employees mentioned above have received injections of polio vaccine . . . and that they have no knowledge of the particular lot being used. It should also be of interest to note that 63 out of the 67 pertinent families eligible for immunization did receive them. These four families who did not participate have the highest integrity."

Habel and Tripp considered the remote possibility that live virus particles in the air were floating into the vaccine during the filling of individual vials. So they called in A. T. Rossano Jr., a specialist in sanitary engineering from Cincinnati. He examined air ducts, flow rates, and wind conditions at the time of filling and concluded that the possibility that live virus was floating into the vaccine was "very remote."

Karl Habel and William Tripp ended their investigation of Cutter Laboratories at noon on May 12, 1955. In a 109-page document submitted to William Workman, they noted several transgressions and made some suggestions, but they knew that none of their findings explained the disaster that had occurred at Cutter Laboratories. They found that prior to February 1955 Cutter had used a concentration of formaldehyde to inactivate virus that was slightly higher than that requested by the federal government. So they recommended exactly a 1 to 4,000 dilution of formaldehyde. They found that the mixing of polio virus with formaldehyde, often done by hand in large, heavy flasks, "may not always be thorough." So they recommended mechanical mixing. They found that in some instances, inactivation of virus occurred at 97 degrees instead of 98 degrees. So they recommended that inactivation be performed in a more consistent manner. They found, like Julius Youngner before them, that live polio virus and inactivated polio vaccine were stored in the same room, but they also found that all containers were sealed. They concluded that "although it might be theoretically desirable to have separate refrigerators for the storage of the virus at all the stages of manufacture, this is not a real point of weakness in the laboratory facilities."

They also found that some of the monkey kidney cells used to grow polio virus were contaminated with a virus called monkey B virus. Monkey B virus occasionally caused mild disease in monkeys but, when inadvertently transmitted to humans, caused severe swelling

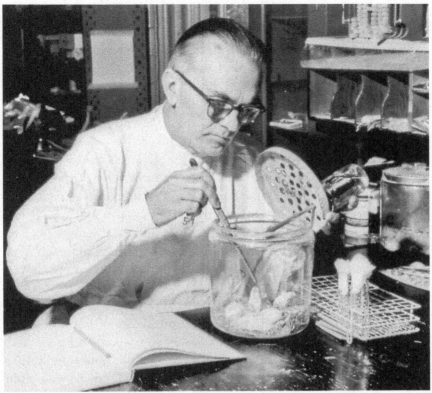

Karl Habel in his laboratory (courtesy of the National Library of Medicine).

of the brain and death; laboratory workers were at particular risk of infection. Cutter had detected the presence of monkey B virus in lots of vaccine prior to shipment, and in every instance lots were appropriately segregated and discarded. (Ironically, years later, Karl Habel accidentally pricked his finger with a specimen obtained from a monkey infected with monkey B virus. As a consequence, he suffered severe, permanent brain damage and was in a coma for many years. He never worked again. "There was a lot of tragedy in this business," said a coworker.) Although Karl Habel knew that something was wrong at Cutter Laboratories, he could not figure out what it was: "I have no explanation as to why cases of polio apparently occurred following use of Cutter's vaccine."

While Habel and Tripp were investigating Cutter Laboratories, a meeting was taking place at the National Institutes of Health (NIH) in Bethesda, Maryland, among pharmaceutical company scientists, polio researchers, and federal officials. The purpose of the meeting was to find out why Cutter was having difficulties inactivating polio virus and why other companies weren't. Federal officials were about to find out that Cutter wasn't the only company having problems.

On Friday, April 29, two days after the first reports of paralysis began to appear and one day after Karl Habel and William Tripp flew to Berkeley, researchers at the NIH began to search for flaws in Cutter's manufacturing protocols. Chaired by NIH director William Sebrell, the meeting included William Workman, Alexander Langmuir, Bernice Eddy, Jonas Salk, James Shannon, and Victor Haas, among others. Sebrell, a nutritionist with no experience in viruses or vaccines, welcomed the participants: "I think all of you know the basic reason why we have called this committee together to discuss and advise us. As of last night we had reports of seven additional cases of polio in vaccinated children in California. All of these cases were vaccinated with Cutter vaccine. . . . We are doing everything that should be done in order to find out what has happened here and why, [and] we want your advice on our procedures as to whether or not they are entirely adequate; and, if they are not, we want to make them so as quickly as possible."

The first day of the meeting, the committee members spent eleven hours reviewing Cutter's protocols, trying to figure out why Cutter had failed. They discussed details of the children paralyzed and killed by Cutter's vaccine. They discussed the specific number of samples tested for live virus during inactivation. They discussed the minimum accepted time of treatment with formaldehyde. They discussed the relative sensitivities of safety tests performed in cell culture and those performed in monkeys. But at the end of the day, there was no clear explanation for why Cutter was having a problem or what Cutter should do differently.

The next day was reserved for presentations by scientists from the pharmaceutical companies. Cutter sent Walter Ward; Parke-Davis sent Bill McLean and Fred Stimpert; Eli Lilly sent Herman Dettwiler; Wyeth sent Robert McAllister; and Sharpe and Dohme (who was starting to make polio vaccine but hadn't distributed it to the public) sent Bettylee Hampil. The expectation was that differences between Cutter's methods of inactivation and those of other companies would show why Cutter was having a problem.

> Walter Ward (Cutter): We have our own problems. We make empirical moves. We will get a fair or good experience for a time and then we get sort of bitten again. We are either awfully unintelligent or there are a number of things here which seem to jump around. It is one of the most difficult things that I personally have ever tackled, and I have felt until now that I have been in on some pretty complicated ones.

This confession surprised no one. The surprise came later.

> Robert McAllister (Wyeth): First, I better say that Wyeth . . . at least for the first few months, had a very rocky road. Between January and April of last year approximately 12 lots passed through the hands of Wyeth Company and, using the 42 tissue culture safety tests, two of these failed, two out of the 12. *However, when the bottle technique was applied, six out of 12 failed.*

By "bottle technique," McAllister was referring to a different kind of tissue culture safety test performed by Wyeth. To detect live virus in polio vaccine, fluid could be inoculated onto small numbers of cells in roller tubes or onto large numbers of cells in bottles. The advantage of bottles was that Wyeth could test larger quantities of vaccine. Wyeth's claim that the bottle technique was more sensitive at detecting live virus worried federal officials in attendance; federal requirements didn't include large-volume safety tests.

The representative from Eli Lilly spoke next:

> Herman Dettwiler (Lilly): Now our experience has been rather varied. We are embarrassed by having gained perhaps too much confidence from our experience last spring [from the field trial]. We put [single]-strained pools on safety tests, mixed the lots immediately, and had the [final vaccine] safety tests running at the same time. *We found a lot of virus in some of them.*

Echoing the presentation by Wyeth's McAllister, Dettwiler admitted that Lilly too had had a problem consistently inactivating virus. Dettwiler went on to say that like Cutter, Lilly found that some safety tests showed no live virus after individual strains were inactivated but did show live virus when these same individual strains were combined for the final vaccine. These inconsistencies again suggested that safety tests were inadequate. Bill McLean's comments added to the uncertainties.

> Bill McLean (Parke-Davis): There is no doubt that this is not a straight line. The curve hills off. We have paid very little attention to the [inactivation] rate. We do it and we draw the line. It usually hits somewhere around 48 to 72 hours. We treat for a period of time in excess of that routine. We rely on safety tests to pick up the approximate 10 percent [of live virus], . . . of those that show up.

McLean was explaining that without a straight line for the rate of inactivation, Parke-Davis was *guessing* at how long to treat with formaldehyde and that about 10 percent of the Parke-Davis lots of final vaccine contained live virus. Salk, silent for most of the meeting, was appalled. He knew that the only way to determine how long to treat polio virus with formaldehyde was to plot the quantities of live virus found during inactivation and to make sure that the line connecting those dots was straight. If it wasn't, it was impossible to determine how long to treat with formaldehyde. Bill McLean said that when they connected the points at Parke-Davis, the line wasn't straight—rather, it started to curve (or, in McLean's words, "hill off"). If the line wasn't straight, then Salk's theoretical trillionfold reduction couldn't occur. Instead of as little as one infectious virus per trillion doses, it was conceivable that live virus could still be present in the vaccine. Worse, given the presentations by Ward, McAllister, Dettwiler, and McLean, it was evident that tissue culture tests weren't particularly sensitive; small quantities of live polio virus contained in the vaccine might not be detected by safety tests.

> "How can you be sure if you do not have a [straight-line] process that you treat it long enough," Salk asked McLean, "and why do you stop at 11 or 14 days?" "Well, you've got to stop sometime," McLean replied.

Hampil described a fundamental problem of polio vaccine manufacture.

> Bettylee Hampil (Sharpe and Dohme): Oh, they are not straight lines. We get nice straight inactivation lines with about 100 [doses] or 150 [doses] of material. But in our bulk they are not straight.

In other words, polio virus could be inactivated fairly easily in relatively small quantities of vaccine, like a few hundred or a few thousand doses, but for large quantities, like a few million doses, the rate of inactivation changed.

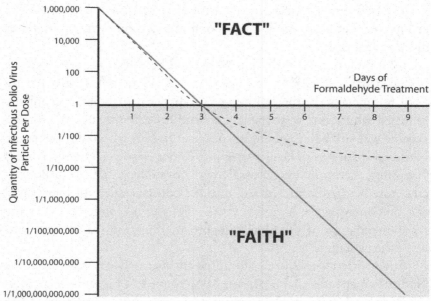

Manufacturers found that they could not duplicate Salk's straight-line theory of inactivation when making large quantities of polio vaccine.

Of all the pharmaceutical company presentations, perhaps the one that unnerved most of those in attendance was that by Parke-Davis's Fred Stimpert.

> Fred Stimpert (Parke-Davis): Let's take the inactivation procedure. Let's say we are doing the best we can. . . . We were having difficulties in irregular safety test reports. . . . We [now observe] our bottles as long as we [can], and if possible, over a 28 day period.

The government required vaccine to be inoculated onto monkey kidney cells, to be observed for fourteen days. If cells still looked healthy, companies could be assured that no live virus was present in the vaccine. But Stimpert said that the fourteen-day safety test could be falsely reassuring; he said that the only way to really know whether live polio virus was contaminating the final vaccine was to observe cells for two more weeks. The data presented by Fred Stimpert meant that vaccine that companies had deemed safe—and vaccine that was approved as safe by the federal government—might still contain live polio virus.

The two-day meeting ended without a clear recommendation. The group considered stopping the polio immunization program but later decided against it.

John Enders, who with Tom Weller and Fred Robbins had won the Nobel Prize in Medicine in 1954, listened to the data presented by Fred Stimpert and others. Enders couldn't accept that government-required safety tests were inadequate and he feared that contaminated vaccine was still being sold to the public. On May 2, two days after the National Institutes of Health meeting, Enders wrote a letter to Sebrell: "I cannot, therefore, longer assert with confidence that the polio vaccine now being distributed and injected consists solely of inactivated and, in consequence, harmless virus. . . . I can no longer approve the recommendation of the Committee to the Surgeon General to continue the program."

Enders's letter to Sebrell prompted another two-day meeting at the National Institutes of Health on May 5 and 6. This time the group decided to ask every manufacturer to stop distributing its vaccine. On May 6 Surgeon General Scheele announced to the press and to the public that all polio vaccinations would be postponed until further notice. Because of Scheele's actions, companies withheld 3.9 million doses of polio vaccine from distribution. The suspension of the polio vaccine program in the United States led to the suspension of similar programs in Great Britain, Sweden, West Germany, and South Africa.

On May 8 Leonard Scheele appeared on television to explain his actions:

> As Surgeon General of the Public Health Service, I recommended the day before yesterday that vaccination programs against polio be temporarily postponed. The decision was based on preliminary reviews of the recommendations of a group of scientists and medical experts who have been consulting with us on the problem that arose when a number of children developed polio after injections with the vaccine of one manufacturer. The review has been completed. . . . Because the Public Health Service believes that every single step in the interest of safety must be taken, we are undertaking, with the help of manufacturers, a reappraisal of all of their tests and processes. This can be thought of, if you like, as a double check. . . . But we believe—and I am sure the American people join us in believing—that in dealing with the lives of our children, it is impossible to be too cautious.

Scheele was walking a fine line. If he told the press the real reason that he had suspended the polio program—that all of the companies were having trouble consistently inactivating polio virus and that safety tests were unreliable—he risked scaring the public away from a vaccine that could save lives. On the other hand, if he withheld information, he risked losing credibility.

One year before, Basil O'Connor had headed a program that had safely inoculated more than four hundred thousand children with Salk's vaccine. Now, in the hands of the federal government, the program was in disarray. O'Connor, unaware of the results of the meeting at the National Institutes of Health and consequently unaware of the problems with other pharmaceutical companies, didn't understand Scheele's logic: "I couldn't understand what he had in mind. Every day he kept saying that the vaccine from the other companies was good, which was true, and now he wanted to put a stop to its use. I told him that the press would knock his head off if some reporter was smart enough to ask how come he was having the manufacturers withdraw a safe vaccine. Naturally, no reporter ever asked the question. Or, if any did, I don't remember Scheele's answer anywhere." Scheele remembered O'Connor's anger and frustration: "Basil O'Connor tried every which way to talk me out of suspending the program. He called me at all hours of the night. He threatened to have me fired."

During the next week William Workman visited all the companies making polio vaccine: Parke-Davis on May 11 and 12, Eli Lilly on May 13 and 14, Wyeth on May 16 and 17, and Pitman-Moore on May 18 and 19. He reviewed and approved specific lots of vaccine so that by May 14, 1 million doses of new vaccine were again distributed to the public. But the review also revealed the exact percentages of vaccine lots made by each pharmaceutical company that were contaminated with live polio virus.

Cutter made 97 lots of individual strains before combining them to make the final vaccine; 21 percent contained live virus. Although all of the lots found to contain live virus were retreated with formaldehyde or destroyed, it was clear that Cutter was having a problem consistently inactivating polio virus. Parke-Davis made 234 lots; 21 percent contained live virus. Eli Lilly made 85 lots; 8 percent contained live virus. Wyeth made 267 lots; 5 percent contained live virus. Pitman-Moore made 126 lots; 2 percent contained live virus. Like Cutter, none of these companies sold vaccine that they knew contained live virus. But it was clear that they were all having trouble inactivating polio virus with formaldehyde.

On May 9 Leonard Scheele made another statement to the press: "I want first and foremost to assure parents of children who have received an injection of polio vaccine this spring that, in the very best judgment of the Public Health Service, they have no cause for alarm." Scheele was reassured because although all the companies had trouble consistently inactivating polio virus, Cutter was the only one that had released a product that caused paralysis and death. Moreover, Karl Habel believed that vaccine that passed safety tests by Cutter was different from vaccine that passed safety tests by other companies: "Other firms . . . may carry out inactivation procedures in such a way that a negative test could quite possibly mean absence of live virus in spite of the lack of sensitivity of the safety test. These differences might then explain the different experience to date in the field between Cutter and other laboratories."

During the next few months, the confidence of Scheele and Habel would be shaken because in the spring of 1955 Cutter Laboratories wasn't the only company to make a vaccine that paralyzed and killed children.

Pamela Erlichman was seven years old when she received a polio vaccine from her school clinic in Bucks County, Pennsylvania. Within days, Pamela couldn't move her left arm, couldn't breathe on her own, and died from polio. Pamela's father, Fulton Erlichman, a local pediatrician, called the school to find out which vaccine his daughter had received. Erlichman knew that Cutter Laboratories distributed small quantities of vaccine in his area, and he assumed that his daughter had received a vaccine from one of its contaminated lots. But Pamela hadn't received Cutter's vaccine. She had received Wyeth's vaccine—lot 236.

When he discovered that his daughter had received Wyeth's, not Cutter's, vaccine, Fulton Erlichman wrote a letter to James Shannon of the National Institutes of Health, requesting a detailed investigation.

"I would be interested in the findings present during the illness and death of my daughter," he wrote. Wyeth's vaccine was already under investigation.

The special unit within Langmuir's Epidemic Intelligence Service that investigated Cutter's vaccine also investigated vaccines made by every other company. The unit, named the Poliomyelitis Surveillance Unit (PSU), was headed by Neal Nathanson. A passionate, quiet, brilliant man, Nathanson had just started a medical residency at the University of Chicago after graduating from Harvard College and Harvard Medical School. On June 10, 1955, after the PSU finished investigating all five companies, it sent its findings to Oveta Culp Hobby, secretary of the Department of Health, Education, and Welfare. The report, entitled *Public Health Service Technical Report on Salk Poliomyelitis Vaccine*, included the exact number of doses of vaccine distributed by each company, the number of cases of polio that followed vaccination, and the number of cases of natural polio expected by chance to follow vaccination.

Between April 15 and May 7 five different companies distributed 4,844,000 doses of polio vaccine throughout the United States. Eli Lilly distributed 2,514,000 doses: twenty-nine cases of polio were reported; twenty-four were expected. Because the number of children expected to get polio by chance alone and the number that actually got polio following Lilly's vaccine were not statistically different and because cases of polio following Lilly's vaccine didn't have the same characteristics as Cutter's cases—such as paralysis in the arm that was inoculated—the PSU concluded that Eli Lilly's vaccine didn't cause paralysis. Parke-Davis distributed 834,000 doses: two cases of polio were reported; three were expected. Pitman-Moore distributed 411,000 doses: two cases were reported; two were expected. Nathanson concluded: "Among the children who received vaccines made by Lilly, Parke Davis, and Pitman-Moore, the numbers of cases reported are within the range expected by chance occurrence."

But Wyeth's vaccine was different. Wyeth distributed 776,000 doses: eleven cases of paralysis followed administration of Wyeth's vaccine—but only two were expected. Nathanson concluded: "The excess of reported cases over the expected number vaccinated with Wyeth product (11 and 2) may be significant, but the numbers are too small to permit firm interpretation of such crude data." One other aspect of the Wyeth cases was worrisome: three children were paralyzed in the inoculated arm. And children immunized with Wyeth's vaccine appeared to be spreading the virus to family members and community contacts, some of whom were also severely paralyzed.

The PSU's preliminary finding spurred further investigation. Between June and August 1955 Neal Nathanson and Alexander Langmuir collected data for a report later entitled *The Wyeth Problem: An Epidemiological Analysis of the Occurrence of Poliomyelitis in Association with Certain Lots of Wyeth Vaccine.* On August 31, 1955, they completed their report. Nathanson began his analysis with a summary of the problem: "During the middle of May a small number of cases were reported to the PSU which raised the question of a possible association with vaccine manufactured by Wyeth Laboratories. Because of the importance of this 'Wyeth Problem' to the broad issue of the safety of polio vaccines, the present report has been prepared. It summarizes in detail the information that has been reported to the PSU in Atlanta. Even now the data are incomplete, but it is possible to give a general description of the epidemiological findings."

Wyeth made four lots of vaccine that were distributed in Maryland, Delaware, Ohio, Pennsylvania, and the District of Columbia—lot numbers 234, 235, 236, and 237. Nathanson determined the number of cases of paralysis that were associated with each lot. He found no cases after lot 234, eight cases after lot 235, twenty-six cases after lot 236, and three cases after lot 237. He concluded that "a situation existed that strongly suggested a causative relation of polio cases with the Wyeth Vaccine lot 236. . . . 21 of 25 total cases reported during the 12-week Study Period were PSU-accepted vaccine-associated cases. Of these . . . 15 were associated with Wyeth Vaccine lot 236. *It is difficult to account for these findings by any other hypothesis than that infective amounts of live virus were present in the vaccine.*" Quietly and with little attention from the public or the media, Wyeth recalled one lot of its vaccine.

The Wyeth Problem was sent to the director of the Communicable Diseases Center, the director of the National Institutes of Health, the Surgeon General of the United States, and the director of the Laboratory of Biologics Control. It was never released to the media, never shown to polio researchers, never shown to the National Foundation, never shown to polio vaccine advisers, never distributed to health care professionals, never published in medical journals, and never made available to defense attorneys in subsequent lawsuits against Cutter Laboratories. As a result, only a handful of people knew about the problem with Wyeth's vaccine.

The author of *The Wyeth Problem,* Neal Nathanson, was twenty-eight years old when he joined Alexander Langmuir at the Communicable Diseases Center. In 1963 Nathanson wrote a landmark series of papers in the *American Journal of Hygiene* describing the Cutter Incident and its cause; these papers remain the single best description of the event. Neal Nathanson's career has now spanned six decades and included important contributions to understanding how and why viruses infect the nervous system. He was chief of the Division of Infectious Diseases at the Johns Hopkins School of Hygiene and Public Health; chairman of the Department of Microbiology at the University of Pennsylvania; and, between 1998 and 2000, director of the Office of AIDS Research at the National Institutes of Health. Although Nathanson published hundreds of papers in medical and scientific journals, the detailed study of Wyeth's polio vaccine is not among them. "The reason it was never submitted for publication was that an administrative decision was made by Alex [Langmuir]," Nathanson recalled, "a decision that was unlikely to have been made in a vacuum."

Nathanson surmised that the government never publicly disclosed the Wyeth problem because it wanted to maintain the public's trust in the polio vaccine program. If people thought that the problem was limited to one company's incompetence, the solution was simply to eliminate that company's vaccine. But if the problem was industry-wide, people would be afraid to use any polio vaccine. "As long as the problem was with one manufacturer and a couple of lots of vaccine," Nathanson recalled, "it would be viewed as an aberration due to sloppy manufacturing or testing procedures and not an intrinsic problem. Once it was extended to a second manufacturer, it would be seen as intrinsic to the product." Also, Cutter simply didn't have the reputation of other companies; it made far fewer products for human use than other companies, and as a consequence, it was far less visible.

Nathanson recalled that "it was a question of Cutter's competence and ethics as compared with other companies such as Wyeth, Pitman-Moore, and Parke-Davis."

David Cutter remembered the perception among Cutter's senior executives that because it was a smaller, lesser known company, it had been singled our unfairly: "I think for the press it was good news. They had somebody to pick on and you can do a lot with that. They had to find some scapegoat, if there was to be one. And I guess it was easier to pick on a company that you'd never heard of, that, therefore, must be a fly-by-night outfit, than it was to pick on the federal government or the biological-science people; because Cutter was virtually an unknown in lay or consumer circles."

When all the data were collected and analyzed, the incidence of paralysis following Cutter's vaccine was tenfold greater than Wyeth's. Although Wyeth had a problem, Cutter's vaccine was by far the most dangerous. During the next two years it would become clear exactly what went wrong at Cutter Laboratories.

6

What Went Wrong at Cutter Laboratories

Show me a hero, and I'll write you a tragedy.
—F. Scott Fitzgerald

A SERIES OF SEVEN EVENTS AT CUTTER LABORA-
tories resulted in a polio vaccine containing live polio virus. For children to be paralyzed and killed, all seven had to occur.

First, Cutter used the Mahoney strain. Jonas Salk had injected
thousands of monkeys to determine which strains of type 1 polio virus
induced the greatest quantities of antibodies, and he found that the
Mahoney strain worked best. When Salk made his choice, he knew
that Mahoney was deadlier than any other type 1 strain, but he felt that
if Mahoney was completely inactivated, it didn't matter. Salk's choice
of the Mahoney strain left pharmaceutical companies little room for
error.

Salk was both right and wrong in choosing the Mahoney strain. If
completely inactivated, it made an excellent vaccine. The Connaught
Medical Research Laboratories at the University of Toronto in Canada
immunized six hundred thousand children safely using inactivated
Mahoney virus, and most vaccine manufacturers still use Mahoney
today. But other type 1 strains far less dangerous than Mahoney also
worked. Using different type 1 strains, Finland, Sweden, Denmark,
England, and the Netherlands dramatically reduced or eliminated polio from their countries.

The government did not require pharmaceutical companies to use
the Mahoney strain. Federal requirements stated that "*any strain* of
each type of virus may be used which produces a vaccine of acceptable potency." If Salk had not chosen Mahoney or if Cutter had chosen a strain other than Mahoney, the Cutter Incident wouldn't have

happened. But all five companies making polio vaccine in the spring of 1955 used Mahoney, so it is hard to fault Cutter for its choice.

Second, Cutter picked a troublesome filtration method. To make the vaccine, polio virus grown in monkey kidney cells was inactivated with formaldehyde. The key step in vaccine production came just after the virus was grown in cells and just before it was inactivated with formaldehyde. Early in his research Salk recognized that monkey kidney cells and cell debris had to be completely and thoroughly removed; if not, polio virus, hidden within the debris, would be protected from formaldehyde. To remove cells and cell debris, Salk recommended Seitz filters, made of thick layers of asbestos. Because Seitz filters were commonly used in the beverage industry, fluids passing through them were often referred to as "gin pure." When Salk first made his vaccine, he used Seitz filters.

Seitz filters were remarkable in their capacity to remove cell debris efficiently and consistently, but filtration times were slow. When Salk was making hundreds of doses of vaccine, a slow method wasn't a problem; but when he made thousands of doses, he needed a faster method. Percival Bazeley, an Australian physician and veterinarian recommended to Salk by the National Foundation, solved the problem. Bazeley, who had a knack for large-scale production because he had recently made large quantities of penicillin in Australia, recommended that to shorten filtration times Salk switch from Seitz filters to glass filters. Glass filters were made by partially fusing heated glass so that it contained holes. Depending on how the glass was fused, the holes were large or small. For vaccine filtration, preparations of virus and cells first passed through coarse glass filters (those with large holes—and then through medium, fine, and ultrafine filters) with smaller and smaller holes. The advantage of glass filters was that filtration times were much faster than with Seitz filters; the disadvantage, in retrospect, was that glass filters occasionally allowed tiny amounts of cell debris to pass through.

In mid-August 1955, four months after the Cutter Incident, Jonas Salk received filtered fluids from several companies. When Salk first looked at these fluids, they appeared to be clear, but when the flasks were "disturbed by a strong swirling motion, the sediment would rise from the center in a tornado-like cone." The sediment observed by

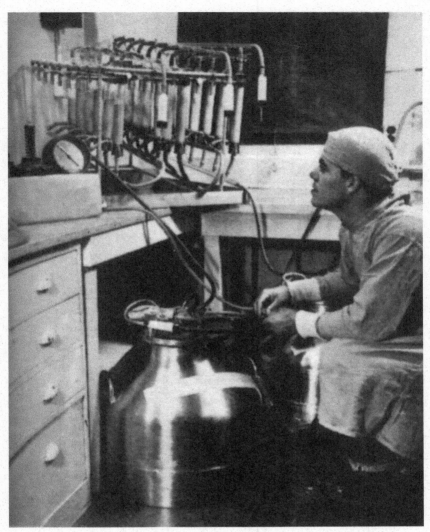

Cutter technician observes the separation of polio virus from cell debris by glass filtration. Inadequate filtration was in large part responsible for the tragedy at Cutter Laboratories (courtesy of the Bayer Corporation).

Salk was cell debris, and it explained why companies were having trouble inactivating virus consistently.

Two years later, at an international polio conference in Geneva, David Bodian, a polio researcher from Johns Hopkins School of Medicine, presented data that helped in part to solve the mystery at Cutter Laboratories. Bodian compared the consistency of inactivation of polio virus from companies that used Seitz filters with that from companies that used glass filters; the results were striking. Companies that used glass filters were thirty-four times more likely to make lots of vaccine that inadvertently contained live virus than companies that used Seitz filters. Bodian said that "the total experience vividly demonstrates the superiority of the method employing Seitz-type filters."

Eli Lilly and Pitman-Moore in the United States and Connaught Laboratories in Canada used Seitz filters and made a vaccine that was safe. But other companies—specifically Parke-Davis, as well as Jonas Salk's laboratory—used glass filters to make safe vaccine. So why did Cutter have the biggest problem? The answer is that glass filters weren't all the same. A. J. Beale supervised the production of polio vaccine for the pharmaceutical giant Glaxo in England. "We made 145 consecutive lots without having any residual polio virus in them," said Beale. "But then there was the retirement of a craftsman at the factory that made the glass. Now glass filters led to a terrible problem and we had live polio virus in the killed polio virus vaccine. We discovered the problem before it was used." Glaxo's experience made it clear that the production of glass filters was an art dependent on the artist. After the retirement of the master craftsman, Glaxo by necessity switched from glass to Seitz filters and never had a problem inactivating polio virus again.

By November 1955, seven months after the Cutter tragedy, the government changed its requirements for making polio vaccine: "Suspensions shall be filtered through a series of filters of efficiency equivalent to that of [a] Seitz type filter pad or two sequential 'ultra-fine' [filters]." David Bodian and A. J. Beale found that Seitz filters were clearly better than glass filters, but their observations weren't made until 1957, two years after the Cutter Incident. In late 1955 the value of Seitz filters and the problem with glass filters were not fully realized. Cutter can't be blamed for using glass filters. But if, like Eli Lilly,

Pitman-Moore, and Connaught, Cutter had chosen to use Seitz filters, the Cutter Incident would not have happened.

Third, safety tests were inadequate. The federal government required two safety tests: vaccine had to be injected into monkeys and inoculated onto monkey kidney cells. If the monkeys weren't paralyzed in thirty days and if the cells didn't die in fourteen days, then vaccine was considered to be free of live polio virus. By the end of April 1955 it was clear that these safety tests were inaccurate.

Soon after the meeting of pharmaceutical company scientists at the National Institutes of Health at the end of April 1955, the government changed its requirements for performing cell culture safety tests. Originally it required that at minimum tissue culture tests be performed using one dose (one-half thimbleful) of vaccine per lot. This regulation meant that companies could test as little as 0.1 percent of the final vaccine for safety. Cutter complied with this requirement. By May 26, 1955, one month after the Cutter Incident, the government changed the requirement to "a sample consisting of at least 1,500 milliliters [about one and one-half quarts] of the final vaccine." It made this change specifically for Cutter Laboratories. Of all the companies, Cutter used the least amount of vaccine to test for safety—one-tenth as much as Lilly. By increasing the quantity of vaccine required for cell culture testing, the government increased the chance of detecting live virus.

Safety tests in monkeys were also inadequate. On June 15, 1955, Carl Eklund, from the United States Public Health Service Laboratory in Hamilton, Montana, took Cutter's production pool number 19468— the pool that had paralyzed and killed schoolchildren in Idaho—and injected it into a monkey. Within several weeks, the monkey was paralyzed. Later Jerome Syverton from the University of Minnesota also found that Cutter's vaccine paralyzed monkeys. Eklund and Syverton had proven that vaccine sold by Cutter Laboratories contained live polio virus. Cutter had tested lot 19468 in monkeys and had found nothing. But Eklund and Syverton did something that Cutter didn't do: they first injected monkeys with cortisone, a steroid. Cortisone weakened the monkeys' immune systems and made them more susceptible to infection. Researchers at the National Institutes of Health further improved safety tests by inoculating vaccine directly into a monkey's spinal cord, a method that was five hundred times more sensitive at detecting live polio virus than inoculation into brain and muscles. As a consequence of these experiments, on September 10, 1955, five months after the Cutter Incident, the government changed requirements to include spinal cord inoculations of cortisone-treated monkeys.

Cutter had complied with government safety tests and had absolute faith in their value—a faith evidenced by one of its pathologists, Donald Trotter. Responsible for monkey safety tests, Trotter knew that some lots of Cutter's vaccine paralyzed monkeys and that other lots of vaccine didn't. Trotter chose to immunize his own children with vaccine that had passed the monkey safety tests. He believed that if a lot of vaccine failed a safety test, then it contained enough live virus to paralyze or kill a monkey, and that if the next lot of vaccine, made by the same people using the same method, passed the test, then it was completely safe.

Cutter was not responsible for the fact that adequate safety tests were not available in the spring of 1955. No company used cortisone-treated monkeys or spinal cord inoculations for safety testing, and only Eli Lilly routinely tested the quantities of vaccine required for cell culture testing months later. Cutter was not at fault, but if better safety tests had been available earlier, the Cutter Incident would not have happened.

Fourth, Cutter let filtered virus sit in the refrigerator for long periods before inactivating it with formaldehyde. Walter Ward and Ralph Houlihan learned how to make polio vaccine for Cutter Laboratories by visiting Jonas Salk's laboratory. At the time of their visits, Salk used glass filters. But Salk's technicians always treated virus with formaldehyde within days of glass filtration; they never let filtered virus sit around. Cutter scientists, in contrast, often left filtered virus in the refrigerator for weeks—and sometimes months—before inactivation with formaldehyde. Among pharmaceutical companies, only Cutter let filtered virus sit around that long. Long periods of storage caused fine clumps of monkey kidney cell debris to form on the bottoms of the flasks. In November 1955 the government changed the requirements: "Within *72 hours* preceding the beginning of inactivation of virus, suspensions shall be filtered through a series of filters." This requirement was prompted solely by the procedures at Cutter Laboratories.

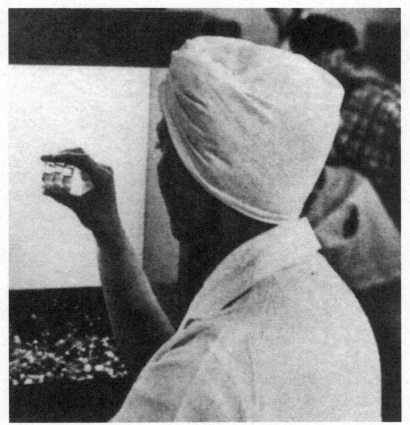

Technician at Cutter Laboratories observes vials of polio vaccine
for clarity; Berkeley, California, 1955 (courtesy of the Bayer
Corporation).

   Fifth and most important, Cutter never constructed a graph to
determine how long to treat polio virus with formaldehyde. Jonas Salk
recommended testing at least four samples during inactivation and
recommended that the last sample be free of live virus. The time that
it took to completely inactivate polio virus with formaldehyde was
determined by the time that it took to eliminate detectable live virus
from one dose of vaccine. If it took three days to eliminate detectable
virus, then the preparation should be treated for an additional six
days—that is, twice the time it took to eliminate virus. The additional
treatment provided the margin of safety that Salk deemed critical to

the production of safe vaccine. Salk clearly stated these guidelines in his publications and in the manufacturing protocol that he prepared for the National Foundation—a protocol that was sent to Cutter Laboratories. Every company that made polio vaccine in the spring of 1955 knew about Salk's theory of inactivation. Although Salk did not provide specific details for how to accomplish complete inactivation, his concepts were clear.

Eli Lilly and Parke-Davis tested six samples during inactivation to determine the length of time it took to inactivate virus; Wyeth tested five samples; Pitman-Moore tested only three samples but always found that detectable virus had been eliminated after seventy-two hours of treatment. Cutter Laboratories never determined when live virus was first eliminated and, therefore, couldn't determine how long to treat with formaldehyde. No company showed a greater disregard for Salk and his theories than Cutter Laboratories. For example, Cutter scientists tested only two samples during the inactivation of lot 19468 (the lot given to schoolchildren in Idaho). After sixteen hours of formaldehyde treatment, 14,500 infectious particles were present; after twenty-eight hours, 38,000 infectious particles were present. The quantity of virus had actually increased. It remains incomprehensible how Walter Ward could look at the inactivation data for lot 19468 and conclude anything other than that he could not reproduce Salk's inactivation results. Ward never showed the inactivation data to his boss, Howard Winegarden, and he never showed them to the head of the company, Robert Cutter. That he chose later to vilify Salk and his technique—Ward always referred to the tragedy at Cutter as "the Salk Incident"—reflects the hubris and isolation of the man. Thirteen years after the tragedy, Robert Cutter fired Walter Ward. Although the reason for his dismissal was never announced, one company executive said that "he wasn't quite the expert he thought he was."

Sixth, Cutter never told other polio researchers that it was having a problem. Cutter knew that its ability to kill polio virus was at best inconsistent (nine of twenty-seven lots had failed safety tests), and it knew that it had done nothing to solve the problem (five of the last seven lots had failed safety tests). Yet when faced with these inadequacies, Cutter Laboratories never told federal regulators of its difficulties and never called the man who was probably best qualified to help—Jonas Salk. Although Walter Ward wrote several letters to Jonas Salk before Cutter sold its vaccine (specifically on January 6, 1955; March 4, 1955; March 31, 1955; and April 4, 1955), he never mentioned his company's difficulties with inactivating polio virus. A call from Ralph Houlihan to Julius Youngner on April 12, 1955—only hours before Cutter distributed its polio vaccine to twenty-six states—was a desperate, pathetic attempt to ask for help. And it was far too late.

Seventh, the federal government didn't know that Cutter Laboratories was having a problem. The National Foundation chose Eli Lilly and Parke-Davis to make vaccine for the field trial because they were the only companies that met the requirement that at least eleven consecutive lots of vaccine pass safety testing. The federal government dropped the consistency requirement when it took over supervision of the polio vaccine program. In consequence, it had no way of knowing that some companies were having trouble inactivating the virus.

Cutter never made eleven consecutive lots of vaccine that passed safety tests. Indeed, it never made four such lots. Later, when asked about the choice to drop the consistency requirement, James Shannon of the National Institutes of Health said that "it was an error of professional judgment." Surgeon General Scheele, in response to the decision to allow companies to withhold from federal regulators information about lots of vaccine that failed safety tests said, "In retrospect, we should have received all the protocols." If the National Foundation's consistency requirement had remained in place after the field trial, the Cutter Incident would not have happened. But again, it is hard to understand how Walter Ward could find that nine of twenty-seven lots of vaccine had failed safety tests and conclude that there was anything other than a fundamental problem with his method of inactivation. Inexplicably, Ward didn't consider production consistency to be important. In a subsequent court case involving Cutter Laboratories, the plaintiff's attorney asked Ward, "In other words, you're saying that you did not follow the theory of production consistency at all when you made a judgment to release your vaccine to the public; is that right?" "This is correct," replied Ward.

Eli Lilly and Parke-Davis each made 15 to 20 lots of vaccine during the field trial. It was not surprising that these two companies made a commercial vaccine that was safe. Of the three remaining companies with less experience (Cutter, Wyeth, and Pitman-Moore), only Pitman-Moore made a commercial vaccine that was safe. Cutter did many things wrong, and it didn't have the internal expertise that was available to other companies. As a consequence, it made a vaccine that was far more dangerous than any other polio vaccine made in the United States or in the world. "They just blindly followed a protocol without thinking about it," recalled a senior virologist at another company. "They didn't have the expertise to think about it."

Cutter Laboratories never blamed itself for the tragedy. The only immediate change in job title was that of Walter Ward, who was asked to head Cutter's operations in Japan. "Nobody was fired and no changes in the company were made," recalled Frank Deromedi, who worked under the direction of Walter Ward. "People did what they were trained and told to do. Nobody had goofed up on anything. There were no errors made. It wasn't something where people necessarily failed when they knew better. They worked on standard procedures on the information that we had received on what the process was supposed to be."

Cutter blamed Jonas Salk for devising a process that was inconsistent, and it blamed the federal government for setting up standards of manufacture and testing that were inadequate. "We made this thing carefully and in accordance with standards set by the government," stated Robert Routh, Frank Deromedi's coworker at Cutter. "This was Salk's process. The NIH approved it. Why are they picking on us? But nobody is blaming the government. Nobody is blaming the NIH for having screwed up and approving a process that didn't work. They were sticking it to us and saying, 'Hey, you guys made the product and you should have known.' How the hell should we have known? It was following a recipe as far as we were concerned."

Many years after the event, Cutter executives still had little understanding of what they had done wrong. Robert Cutter, when asked why his company had more trouble than other companies, said, "Most of the others had deaths from the vaccine, but on a much smaller scale than did Cutter, because we were the 'firstest with the mostest.' We produced and delivered more vaccine in the early states than did any other manufacturer." But Cutter wasn't the first with the most. Although six of the original thirteen lots of vaccine licensed by the government were made by Cutter Laboratories, between April 15 and May 7, 1955, Eli Lilly released 2.5 million doses, Parke-Davis released 830,000 doses, Wyeth released 776,000 doses, Pitman-Moore released 410,000 doses, and Cutter released 380,000 doses. Cutter actually made the least vaccine. And contrary to Robert Cutter's assertions, most other companies didn't make vaccines that killed children. Only Wyeth made such a vaccine; and the incidence of paralysis and death following Wyeth's vaccine was far lower than Cutter's.

Walter Ward and Howard Winegarden also never understood what happened at Cutter. Winegarden, the director of research for Cutter in 1955, recalled the following: "From one of the lots of vaccine that later on gave us plenty of trouble in Idaho, 10,000 doses were used in New Mexico or Arizona and they had no problems. The answer probably was that those people had had polio epidemics off and on for years. There was a higher level of natural immunity than you had in Idaho, for example. That seems to be the answer right there. So, you see, we had no way of knowing we were doing anything wrong. We thought we were doing a fine job. Of course, the other companies all had trouble. We got most of the publicity, but they had trouble too." Winegarden and Ward were right: the number of children paralyzed by Cutter's vaccine in New Mexico and Arizona was about one-tenth of that in Idaho. But the number of children immunized in New Mexico and Arizona was also about one-tenth of that in Idaho, so the *incidence* of paralysis caused by Cutter's vaccine was the same in all three states. Children in Idaho were not more susceptible to polio than children from other states; they were paralyzed and killed because they were given a vaccine that was highly contaminated with live polio virus.

On June 22 and 23, 1955, two months after the Cutter Incident, Tennessee Democrat Percy Priest chaired a congressional hearing to determine who was responsible for the tragedy. The committee, and those who testified before it, variously blamed the National Foundation for Infantile Paralysis, Congressman Richard Nixon, the Laboratory of Biologics Control, and Jonas Salk.

The National Foundation was in charge of the polio vaccine program from 1932 to 1955; it had supervised the research, development, manufacture, and testing of the vaccine. On April 12, 1955, the foundation passed the baton to the federal government. After the Cutter Incident, many physicians, scientists, professional organizations, public health officials, and politicians felt that the National Foundation had rushed the research, staged a clinical trial of a vaccine that wasn't ready, and forced the government to license a product that lacked adequate safety tests. Columnist Walter Lippmann of the New York *Herald Tribune,* who founded the political weekly the *New Republic* and whose column was syndicated in 250 newspapers, criticized the foundation for staging a show at Ann Arbor that duped the public: "There are those who have had great misgivings ever since April 12 [1955] about the dramatic buildup, the theatrical suspense, and the spectacular publicity with which the effectiveness of the Salk vaccine was proclaimed. It was more like announcing the results of an election than the results of a scientific inquiry. . . . For the public the proof that polio had been conquered was . . . in the elaboration of the show, the eminence of the actors, the high-powered publicity itself." An editorial in the *New England Journal of Medicine,* a publication of the Massachusetts Medical Society, also criticized the foundation: "In the final analysis it is physicians who must assume some of the responsibility for allowing themselves to be drafted by methods of the modern impresario into a scientific version of grand opera."

At the congressional hearing Basil O'Connor defended himself and his foundation by subtly laying the tragedy at the feet of the government: "So long as the Salk vaccine and its research were in the hands of the National Foundation, you had some intelligence, intellectual integrity, and total courage—and you had no politics whatsoever." It is hard to argue with O'Connor's logic. The National Foundation spent more money on polio research than any other foundation or government in the world—and it got what it paid for. In a period of slightly more than twenty years, the foundation had helped determine how many types of polio caused disease, how polio virus was spread from one person to another, how polio virus traveled to the spinal cord, how polio antibodies protected against disease, and how polio virus could be grown in cell culture. By supporting the laboratory of Jonas Salk, the foundation had determined how to kill polio virus, which strains of polio virus were best able to induce polio antibodies, and which strains best protected monkeys—and eventually children—from the disease. Basil O'Connor was not in charge of deciding which researchers should be funded and what those researchers should study—those tasks were in the hands of the National Foundation's Immunization Committee, a group that consisted of Thomas Rivers, Jonas Salk, John Enders, Joe Smadel, William McDowell Hammon, Howard Shaughnessey, Albert Sabin, and others. It was not possible for the foundation to have collected a group of advisers better informed or more highly regarded than the members of the Immunization Committee. Because of the National Foundation, the polio vaccine trial performed in the United States in 1954 was the most thorough and best organized of its day. More than 1.8 million children participated in the trial, and in the end, an inactivated polio vaccine was found to be safe and effective. Without the National Foundation, the development of a polio vaccine would have been infinitely slower. Despite its Madison Avenue style of promoting disease awareness, the National Foundation was not to blame for the Cutter tragedy.

Politicians blamed other politicians. At Priest's congressional hearing Arthur Klein, a Democratic congressman from New York City, said, "I have heard charges made, and they are fairly current in Washington. . . . The story that I heard is that a very, very prominent politician from California brought pressure on Mrs. Hobby, the Secretary of the Department [of Health, Education, and Welfare], with regard to licensing Cutter Laboratories." Klein was accusing Richard Nixon, then Vice President, of influencing Hobby to license a vaccine made by Cutter, a California company. Hobby, who appeared before the committee the next day, responded to Klein's accusations: "There is no politics in this. No person ever attempted to bring undue pressure on me at any time in the 30 months I have been on the job." Hobby, who knew little about medicine, science, vaccines, or vaccine manufacture, was not involved in the decision by the Laboratory of Biologics Control to license the polio vaccine. Therefore, political pressure on Hobby couldn't have influenced the decision to license Cutter's vaccine. Although Richard Nixon was responsible for a great many things, the Cutter Incident wasn't one of them.

The agency that suffered the brunt of the criticism—and the one that was most affected by the Cutter tragedy—was the Laboratory of

Biologics Control. During the Priest hearings, Senator Estes Kefauver from Tennessee said: "There is no excuse whatever for starting and stopping, scaring everyone to death. . . . It is one of the worst bungled programs I have ever seen." Senator Wayne Morse of Oregon lamented, "The federal government inspects meat in the slaughterhouses more carefully than it has inspected the polio vaccine."

For their roles in the Cutter Incident, almost everyone involved in regulating vaccines was fired. Ruth Kirchstein, formerly director of the National Institute of General Medical Services within the National Institutes of Health, was in 1957 a researcher involved in the regulation of polio vaccines. She recalled the somber mood of the vaccine regulators following the Cutter Incident: "When Cutter came, every person who had anything to do with that vaccine was fired; every single person all the way up, because the government took full responsibility for it. Bill [Workman] lost his job as lab chief. He was a government civil servant so he didn't lose his salary. Above Workman was the director of the National Microbiological Institute, Victor Haas. Above him was the director of the National Institutes of Health, William Sebrell. Above him was the Surgeon General, Leonard Scheele. And above him was Secretary Hobby. All were fired. Every one of them lost their jobs. It was the usual thing. If the federal government gets caught, everybody involved has to leave." Perhaps the man most affected by the tragedy was the man most responsible for licensing the vaccine, William Workman. "He was put off in a corner somewhere and retired five years later," remembered Kirchstein. "He was a broken man."

The federal government was accountable for two big changes from the 1954 field trial run by the National Foundation (where more than four hundred thousand children had been inoculated safely) and the 1955 commercial vaccine program (where Cutter and Wyeth made vaccines that paralyzed and killed children). First, it dropped the consecutive-lot requirement. For the field trial, Eli Lilly and Parke-Davis were required to make eleven consecutive lots of vaccine that passed safety tests. With this consecutive-lot requirement, Lilly and Parke-Davis learned to make safe vaccines quickly. If the consecutive-lot requirement had remained in place in 1955, neither Cutter nor Wyeth would have been allowed to participate in the program. Second, the government did not examine protocols for lots of vaccine that had failed safety tests. The National Foundation examined every protocol from every lot of vaccine made for the field trial. If the Laboratory of Biologics Control had done the same, the government would have known that Cutter couldn't consistently inactivate virus; moreover, looking at every protocol would not have required additional resources or personnel. The Laboratory of Biologics Control also ignored the warnings of Bernice Eddy five months before licensure that Cutter was having trouble inactivating polio virus. Eddy's pleas were lost in the noise that Parke-Davis and Lilly had also had problems inactivating virus when they first started to make their vaccines. The federal government, through its vaccine regulatory agency, the Laboratory of Biologics Control, was in the best position to avoid the Cutter tragedy.

In June 1955 Jonas Salk was one of the few scientists in the world who believed in his straight-line theory of virus inactivation. At the Priest congressional hearings scientists weighed in with their criticisms of Salk. Two of them were Nobel laureates, Wendell Stanley and John Enders. Stanley, winner of the Nobel Prize in Chemistry in 1946 for his work on viral proteins, rejected Salk's straight-line theory: "Eventually what is taking place here is a chemical reaction, a combination between formaldehyde and polio virus. . . . The chemist will tell you that in such a reaction it is *theoretically impossible to wind up with a situation in which you have no active virus.*" Enders, who won the Nobel Prize in Medicine in 1954, also didn't believe in Salk or his theories: "There has been some doubt cast on the process of inactivation of the virus. We do not know absolutely whether it works according to theory." In front of Congress, the media, the nation, and the world, John Enders, William McDowall Hammon, and Albert Sabin voted to stop Salk's vaccine. Privately, Enders was less politic. At a government meeting in May he leaned across the table and, while staring at Salk, said, "It is quack medicine to pretend that this is a killed vaccine when you know that it has live virus in it. Every batch has live virus in it." Salk, usually stoic in the face of his detractors, later recalled, "That was the first and only time in my life that I felt suicidal. There was no hope, no hope at all."

Through the later part of 1955 and all of 1956, 100 million doses of polio vaccine were given without incident. In 1957 David Bodian concluded that "inactivation data of manufacturers throughout the world show beyond a doubt that the inactivation rate of polio virus, as established by Salk, is sufficiently approximate to a straight line" and that "completely satisfactory inactivation can be obtained by means of the present method of inactivation." Between 1956 and 1961, 400 million doses of Salk's polio vaccine were administered in the United States without causing a single case of paralysis. Jonas Salk and his straight-line theory of inactivation were not to blame for the Cutter tragedy.

On May 14, 1955, the federal government released 1 million doses of polio vaccine. According to Surgeon General Scheele, vaccine was "double-checked" to make sure that it was safe, but parents were confused. An article in *The New York Times* described the dilemma: "The nation is now badly scared. Never before have reports of the number of polio cases been so widely publicized and so carefully studied. Millions of parents fear that if their children don't get the vaccine they may get polio, but if they get the vaccine, it might give them polio."

Leonard Scheele and public health officials said that the vaccine was safe. But several polio researchers said that it wasn't. Further, the American Academy of Pediatrics sent the following statement to every pediatrician in the United States: "In view of the difficulties which have arisen with respect to the manufacture, testing, and usage of large volumes of polio vaccine . . . the American Academy of Pediatrics recommends that injections of this vaccine be *discontinued* for the present." Scheele, by recommending the polio vaccine soon after it had paralyzed many children, was forcing parents to reconcile two irreconcilable notions: that a child should receive only a vaccine that was safe and that (given that medicine is always a process of evolution) future vaccines were likely to be safer. In a report to Oveta Culp Hobby, Scheele said that "we must weigh potential benefits against possible hazards." Scheele was saying that the question wasn't "When was a vaccine good?" but "When was it good enough?" Parents now had to weigh the risks of their children getting paralyzed by polio against the possibility of their getting paralyzed by the polio vaccine. This wasn't the first time that people were frightened by a harmful vaccine.

The first vaccine that had caused concern was the first vaccine ever used. Benjamin Franklin, lamenting the loss of his son to smallpox, wrote "I lost one of my sons, a fine boy of four years old, by the small-pox, taken in the common way. I long regretted bitterly, and still regret, that I had not given it to him by inoculation. This I mention for the sake of parents who omit that operation, on the supposition that they should never forgive themselves if a child died under it; my example showing the regret may be the same either way." Franklin regretted not giving the smallpox vaccine to his son. But Franklin's son died in 1736, sixty years before Edward Jenner developed his smallpox vaccine from cows—and thirteen years before Jenner was born. What was Benjamin Franklin talking about?

In 1670 Edward Wortley Montagu was Britain's ambassador to the Ottoman Empire. His wife, Lady Mary Montagu, was familiar with smallpox; she watched her brother die from it and was herself disfigured by the disease. When she arrived in Constantinople, she found to her surprise that smallpox could be prevented. Crusts were taken from patients recovering from smallpox, ground up, and rubbed into cuts, scratches, or opened veins. The process, called "inoculation" (from the Latin *inoculare*, "to graft"), was a common practice. In the seventeenth century it was clear that those who survived smallpox didn't get infected again. People reasoned that crusts taken from recovering patients might cause a weaker but protective form of the disease.

On April 1, 1717, Lady Montagu wrote a letter to a friend: "The small-pox so fatal and so general among us, is here entirely harmless by the invention of ingrafting, which is the term they give it. There is a set of old women who perform the operation. People make parties for this purpose, and when they are met, the old woman comes with a nut-shell full of the matter of the best sort of small-pox, and asks you what vein you please to have opened. She immediately rips open that you offer her with a large needle and puts into the vein as much matter as can lay upon the head of her needle, and after that binds up the little wound; and in that manner opens four or five veins. Every year thousands undergo this operation; they take the small-pox here by way of diversion, as they take the waters in other countries."

When Lady Mary returned to England, she brought the inoculation process with her. In the spring of 1721, during an outbreak of smallpox in London, an experiment was performed to test Lady

Mary's inoculation. With freedom as their reward, six condemned criminals at Newgate Prison (three men and three women) volunteered to participate; on August 9, 1721, they were inoculated. Following the inoculation, one woman, Elizabeth Harrison, returned to Hertford, where she slept in a bed next to a ten-year-old boy with severe smallpox. Harrison never got smallpox. Later, after larger experiments were performed, the Royal Society in London concluded that the inoculation was effective in preventing smallpox, and in 1745 the London Smallpox and Inoculation Hospital was founded.

News of the inoculation spread. Cotton Mather, a Puritan clergyman in Boston, encouraged its use. During a smallpox epidemic in Boston in 1721—when half of the city's residents were infected with smallpox—the death rate was one in six for those who were not inoculated but only one in forty-seven for those who were inoculated. But there were risks. Because the vaccine contained live human smallpox, some people died from the inoculation; for example, the death of the two-year-old son of the Earl of Sunderland was highly publicized in London. But despite the high risks, Benjamin Franklin regretted his lost opportunity.

The next vaccine that frightened parents was the one developed by Louis Pasteur to prevent rabies. Made from rabbit nervous tissue, rabies vaccine occasionally caused severe neurological complications like paralysis and seizures; the incidence of such reactions was as high as 1 in every 230 immunized people. Because the incidence of death from rabies was 100 percent, the decision to give rabies vaccine to a child bitten by a rabid animal was an easy one. But for parents whose children were bitten by an animal that couldn't be found—and might or might not have rabies—the choice was much harder. It took more than one and one-half centuries for rabies vaccine to be made in tissues that did not contain nerve cells. By the early 1970s rabies vaccines made from human embryo (fetal) cells eliminated the risk of paralysis and seizures.

Another vaccine that precipitated panic was the one for yellow fever, given to American soldiers in 1942. By the early 1940s the vaccine contained a stabilizer, human serum, to protect the vaccine virus from changes in temperature. Unfortunately, one of the people who donated serum for use in the vaccine had hepatitis. At the time that the serum was collected, scientists didn't know that there were different types of hepatitis viruses (such as hepatitis A, B, and C); also, it wasn't clear how hepatitis spread through the body or how it was transmitted from one person to another. In March 1942 the Surgeon General's Office noted a striking increase in the number of military personnel with hepatitis; fifty thousand soldiers given the contaminated yellow fever vaccine had developed hepatitis, and sixty-two died from the disease. A study forty-five years later estimated that as many as three hundred thirty thousand soldiers had been inadvertently infected with what we now know was hepatitis B virus. Human serum was never used as a vaccine stabilizer again. Different stabilizers, such as sorbitol and gelatin, are now used, and people immunized with yellow fever vaccine no longer risk infection from hepatitis B virus. But for soldiers traveling in the mid-1940s to areas of the world where yellow fever was common, the fear of the vaccine probably outweighed the fear of the disease.

The worst vaccine disaster occurred in Lubeck, Germany, in the early 1900s. In 1921 two French researchers, Léon Calmette, a physician, and Camille Guérin, a veterinarian, developed a vaccine to prevent tuberculosis, which was caused by a bacterium called *Mycobacterium tuberculosis*. Calmette and Guérin reasoned that they could take a similar bacterium from cows—*Mycobacterium bovis*—weaken it by serially growing it in broth, and use it as a vaccine. They called their vaccine BCG (Bacillus of Calmette and Guérin), a modified form of which is still used today.

In 1929, 250 ten-day-old children in Lubeck were fed a BCG vaccine that unfortunately wasn't made of BCG. The laboratory that made the vaccine mistakenly grew *Mycobacterium tuberculosis* in the broth instead of *Mycobacterium bovis*. As a consequence, babies were inoculated with massive quantities of live, highly lethal tuberculosis bacteria; seventy-two infants died as a result of the mistake. Nothing was learned from the Lubeck disaster. Techniques to differentiate BCG from *Mycobacterium tuberculosis* were already available, and the two bacteria were easily distinguished when grown in the laboratory (they were different colors). It was a fatal and preventable laboratory error that was never repeated. All but two countries in the world—the United States and the Netherlands—have routinely given BCG vaccine to infants.

During the summer of 1955, two to three months after the recall of Cutter's vaccine, polio epidemics swept across the United States. Doctors, public health officials, and polio experts were divided; some recommended the vaccine and others didn't. Outbreaks in Massachusetts and Illinois revealed which recommendation was the right one.

During the first week of July 1955 an outbreak of polio began in Boston and spread throughout Massachusetts; polio paralyzed more than seventeen hundred people. For those who never received Salk's polio vaccine, the incidence of infection was one per five hundred residents. For those who received one dose of polio vaccine, the incidence was one per one thousand, and for those who received two doses, the incidence was one per two thousand. People who were not vaccinated were four times more likely to get polio than those who were vaccinated.

In Illinois the value of the polio vaccine was also clear. Beginning on June 21, 1955, an outbreak of polio in Chicago paralyzed more than eight hundred people. The outbreak lasted for four months and was the second largest in the city's history. For those who chose not to receive Salk's vaccine, the incidence of infection was seventy-six per one hundred thousand; for those who received one dose, the incidence was thirty per one hundred thousand; for those who received two doses, the incidence was seven per one hundred thousand; and for those who received the recommended three doses, the incidence was zero per one hundred thousand. Salk's vaccine, if used as recommended, completely protected against paralysis. Thirty-six people died in Chicago that summer from polio; none had received all three doses of Salk's vaccine.

Ironically the Cutter Incident—by creating the perception among scientists and the public that Salk's vaccine was dangerous—led in part to the development of a polio vaccine that was more dangerous.

In the years following the licensure of Salk's polio vaccine, the number of polio victims declined dramatically. Between 1950 and 1954 polio paralyzed fifteen of every one hundred thousand people in the United States. But between 1955 and 1961, after 400 million doses of Salk's vaccine had been used, the incidence of paralysis was two per one hundred thousand—a decrease of almost 90 percent. Salk's vaccine worked, but because of the Cutter Incident, many feared that safety tests still weren't sensitive enough to detect small quantities of live polio virus. Scientists and public health officials decided to substitute something perceived as risky (the Salk vaccine) with something that would prove to be riskier (the Sabin vaccine).

Albert Sabin wanted to make a vaccine that provided better immunity than Salk's vaccine. He also wanted to make a vaccine that wasn't dependent on the relative abilities of different pharmaceutical companies to inactivate polio virus. Born in Bialystok, Russia, Sabin trained in medicine at New York University and in virology at the Rockefeller Institute. At once charismatic, egotistical, erudite, and vindictive, Sabin was determined to defeat Salk and his vaccine. To make his vaccine, Sabin took the three strains of natural polio virus—types 1, 2, and 3— and grew them in monkey kidney or testicular cells over and over again. As the viruses grew better and better in monkey cells, they became less and less capable of growing in people and causing disease. Sabin tested his live weakened polio vaccine in 90 million people in Russia; 75 million were inoculated in only one year.

In 1961 the United States was poised to abandon Salk's vaccine in favor of Sabin's, but there was one problem. In 1957 George Dick, a young professor of microbiology at Queen's University in Belfast, Ireland, found something alarming. Dick took a live weakened polio virus and inoculated it into the brains of 12 monkeys; none were paralyzed. Then he took the vaccine, fed it to 170 young children, collected their feces, and administered the vaccine virus that was shed in their feces back into the brains of monkeys. This time 11 of 22 monkeys were paralyzed. Somehow, the weakened polio virus had regained its ability to cause paralysis as it passed through children's intestines. Dick concluded: "The laboratory characteristics of attenuation shown by [the weakened vaccine] which made it appear suitable for trial as a vaccine *are not maintained after multiplication in human gut*"; he warned that performing a large-scale vaccine trial with live weakened polio viruses could be dangerous. Dick's warning was an ominous predictor of future events.

In 1962 the United States faced the choice of continuing to use Salk's killed polio vaccine or switching to Sabin's live weakened viral vaccine. Sabin's vaccine was more attractive for several reasons. It protected 100 percent of children from polio, as compared with about 80 percent inoculated with Salk's vaccine. It was much easier to make and cost only thirty cents per dose—five times less expensive than Salk's vaccine. It protected people who were in contact with vaccinated children. Sabin's vaccine viruses, because they multiplied many times in the intestines, were often spread from one person to another. Twenty-five percent of people who came in close contact with someone given Sabin's vaccine developed polio antibodies even though they hadn't been immunized (this was called "contact immunity"). Because immunization rates in the United States were low, the spread of vaccine viruses from one person to another was considered desirable. And it was easy to give. Drops of the vaccine put on sugar cubes were readily accepted by children; unlike Salk's vaccine, Sabin's didn't require a needle, a syringe, or a trained nurse.

But Sabin's vaccine had one big disadvantage: it was unstable. An advisory committee to the surgeon general of the United States in 1961 stated that one of the three strains in Sabin's vaccine (type 3) "shows a tendency to change its [ability to cause paralysis] after passage in man" and urged that a "superior type 3 strain" be sought. But a better type 3 vaccine was never made, and in 1962 the United States switched from Salk's vaccine to Sabin's.

On October 5, 1964, after 100 million doses of Sabin's polio vaccine had been distributed in the United States, an article appeared in the *Journal of the American Medical Association* confirming George Dick's observations and the advisory committee's worst fears. Not only was Sabin's vaccine paralyzing monkeys after passing through children's intestines, it was also paralyzing people. Fifty-seven cases of paralysis occurred following Sabin's vaccine; thirty-six were caused by type 3 polio virus. Cases of paralysis were not associated with any particular lot of vaccine or with a vaccine made by one company. The chance that thirty-six people had been coincidentally infected with natural type 3 polio virus following Sabin's vaccine—and hadn't actually been paralyzed by Sabin's type 3 vaccine virus—was 185 million to 1. Despite these odds, Sabin refused to believe the results. "I cannot accept the conclusion of this report," he said.

Between 1964 and 1979 Sabin's vaccine was dropped onto sugar cubes and given to millions of children in the United States. Public health officials knew that Sabin's vaccine caused paralysis, but they reasoned that because paralysis was rare (one of seven hundred fifty thousand immunized children was paralyzed after the first dose), the benefits of the vaccine outweighed its risks. By 1979 paralysis caused by natural polio virus was completely eliminated from the United States—a remarkable achievement. Although paralysis caused by natural polio virus was eliminated by Sabin's vaccine, paralysis caused by Sabin's vaccine wasn't eliminated; every year in the United States between 1980 and 1996, six to eight children were paralyzed by Albert Sabin's vaccine viruses.

Jonas Salk knew that his vaccine was better. In the late 1970s in a letter to Alexander Langmuir, Salk pleaded for the government to switch back to his vaccine. He argued that not one case of paralysis caused by a polio vaccine "should be regarded as acceptable if avoidable." Eighteen years passed before the United States switched back to Jonas Salk's vaccine; during that time another two hundred people were paralyzed by Sabin's vaccine. On October 20, 1998, the Advisory Committee for Immunization Practices—the principal body that advises the federal government about vaccine use—recommended to the Centers for Disease Control and Prevention that children use Salk's vaccine exclusively. Sabin's polio vaccine is no longer available in the United States.

Jonas Salk died on June 23, 1995, three years before the United States considered his vaccine to be the last, best vaccine to prevent polio. On the world's stage, Salk was a respected figure. In a survey conducted in 1958, Salk was regarded as one of the two best-known living American scientists; Robert Oppenheimer, the developer of the atomic bomb, was the other. But many of his colleagues dismissed Salk as a lightweight or a fake. No one was more critical, more mean spirited, or more persistent in his attacks than Albert Sabin. A member of the debate team in college, Sabin routinely and consistently humiliated Salk in public.

In 1948, after John Enders figured out how to grow polio virus in monkey cells, an article appeared in a publication by the National Foundation claiming that large quantities of formaldehyde-killed polio virus might soon be available to protect children against polio. Albert Sabin took exception to this article and wrote a letter to Basil O'Connor: "Even if the need for large quantities of virus could be met," said Sabin, "there is no valid reason for believing at this time that 'killed virus' vaccines can be of any practical value." Sabin's campaign to discredit the formaldehyde-inactivated polio vaccine, and later to discredit Jonas Salk, had begun.

In 1953, after Salk presented his studies of children at the Watson and Polk facilities—studies that caused the media to express hope that an inactivated polio vaccine might work—Sabin, addressing a scientific meeting in New York City, said, "Since there is an impression that a practicable vaccine for poliomyelitis is either at hand or immediately around the corner, it may be best to start this discussion with the statement that such a vaccine is not now at hand and that one can only guess as to whether it is around the corner." Later that year, in front of a congressional committee, Sabin again opposed the growing acceptance of Salk and his vaccine: "I, for one, would strongly oppose large-scale tests of tens of thousands or hundreds of thousands of children based on the work of any one investigator." In 1954, after Salk presented more data showing that his vaccine worked and after *Life* magazine published a story detailing Salk's achievements, Sabin stood in front of scientists at the Michigan Medical Society and said, "I felt certain that after you all had read the *Life* magazine story of the conquest of polio, no one would be here. Let us not confuse optimism with achievement."

Prior to the field trial, when Walter Winchell said that the government was preparing "little white coffins" for children expected to die during the trial of Salk's vaccine, Sabin failed to stand up for his colleague. "The field study is premature," he said. When Henry Kempe of the University of California, San Francisco, wrote a letter to the American Academy of Pediatrics opposing its endorsement of the upcoming field trial, Sabin wrote a letter supporting Kempe's objections: "I completely agree with [Kempe's] conclusion 'that the formalin-inactivated vaccine is insufficiently tested for mass trial, potentially unsafe, of undetermined potency, and of undetermined stability.'" Sabin then sent a copy of his letter to Salk with a note attached: "Dear Jonas, This is for your information—so that you'll know what I am saying behind your back. This incidentally is also the opinion of many others whose judgment you respect. 'Love and Kisses' are being saved up. Albert." On March 26, 1953, before his radio address to the nation prior to the field trial, Salk sent a copy of his prepared text to Sabin for review. "He phoned me, incensed," recalled Salk. "Told me I was misleading the public. Urged me not to do it. I was flabbergasted."

In 1970 Richard Nixon awarded the National Medal of Science to Sabin. He lauded Sabin for his "numerous fundamental contributions to the understanding of viruses and viral diseases, culminating in the development of the vaccine which has eliminated poliomyelitis as a major threat to human health." Sabin, picking up on Nixon's phrasing, later said, "I developed *the* vaccine, not *a* vaccine."

At the age of eighty-four, three years before his death, Albert Sabin fired one parting shot at Jonas Salk. "It was pure kitchen chemistry," said Sabin. "Salk didn't discover anything." Despite Sabin's vigorous objections about the safety, potency, and effectiveness of Salk's vaccine, it was Sabin's vaccine that came with the high price of paralysis—a price that was independent of which company made it and that was paid by every country that used it.

Sabin's attacks on Jonas Salk were the most direct and the most personal, but many scientists didn't believe that Salk or his work deserved special recognition. Polio researchers such as John Paul, Joseph Smadel, John Enders, Thomas Weller, Frederick Robbins, David Bodian, Albert Sabin, and Thomas Rivers were all elected to the National Academy of Sciences, a prestigious society for those who make important contributions to science. But Salk was never elected. Scientists and voting members of the academy claimed that Salk hadn't done anything original. Thomas Rivers, when asked why Salk was never elected into the academy, said, "Original work! You don't get into the Academy without [doing] original work! Just as you don't get the Nobel

Prize except for original work. Now, I'm not saying that Jonas wasn't a damned good man, but there had been killed vaccines before. Lots of them. And formalin-killed ones at that." Thomas Weller, co-winner of the Nobel Prize with John Enders, said, "Salk wasn't elected to the National Academy of Sciences because he just wasn't a very good scientist." Renato Dulbecco, winner of the Nobel Prize in Medicine in 1975 for his work on viruses that cause cancer, wrote Salk's obituary for the scientific journal *Nature:* "For his work on polio vaccine, Salk received every major recognition available in the world from the public and governments. But he received no recognition from the scientific world—he was not awarded the Nobel Prize, nor did he become a member of the U.S. National Academy of Sciences. The reason is that he did not make any innovative scientific discovery."

What did Jonas Salk discover? Salk wasn't the first person to make a polio vaccine by inactivating a virus with formaldehyde (that was Maurice Brodie); he wasn't the first person to figure out how to grow polio virus in cell culture (that was John Enders); and he wasn't the first person to give inactivated polio virus to monkeys or to children (Johns Hopkins researchers did that). But Jonas Salk was the first to do many things. He was the first to prove that several doses of his killed viral vaccine induced polio antibodies at levels similar to those found after natural infection. He called this phenomenon "immunologic memory." Before Salk's observation, scientists thought that only natural infections or live weakened vaccine viruses could do this. Salk's concept of immunologic memory is now understood at the molecular level, but at the time it represented a dramatic change in thinking. For this observation alone, Salk should have been awarded the Nobel Prize.

Salk was the first to develop a method to inactivate polio virus in a controlled and reproducible manner. Maurice Brodie and the Johns Hopkins researchers had inactivated polio virus with formaldehyde. But Salk found that using his straight-line theory of inactivation, he could efficiently and quantitatively separate the ability of polio virus to induce protective antibodies from its ability to induce disease. The straight-line theory is still used today to determine how long to inactivate polio virus.

Salk was the first to introduce the notion of progressive filtration as a method to separate cells and cellular debris from polio virus before inactivation. This technique was vital to the production of a virus that was fully susceptible to the effects of formaldehyde.

Finally, Salk, in collaboration with his coworker Julius Youngner, was the first to develop methods to determine the quantity of polio virus in cell culture and the quantity of polio antibodies in blood. Using these techniques, Salk and Youngner picked three strains of polio for their vaccine. These same three strains are used to make inactivated polio vaccines today.

Dulbecco, in his obituary of Salk, also noted the following: "Salk's research met many of the characteristics of good science, such as independence, originality in the pursuit of an unpopular goal, and ability to conclude successfully a project in which no one else believed. His dedication was complete and totally unselfish. It is true that he did not contribute any technological advance; but is science only technology?" Although not appreciated by many scientists, Salk made several important conceptual and technological advances that led to one of the greatest public health achievements of our time.

Cutter in Court

Often with Belli you had a media circus. You just walked down the street and you had a media circus.
—Richard Gerry of the law firm of Belli, Ashe, and Gerry

IN 1996 A CARTOON IN THE *SAN DIEGO UNION Tribune* depicted St. Peter on the telephone. Standing before him, smiling like an angel, was a well-dressed man: "I've got a guy here claiming he was struck and injured by one of the Pearly Gates," said St. Peter. Inscribed on the man's briefcase was the name "M. Belli."

From the 1950s through the 1990s Melvin Belli was one of the most influential lawyers in the United States. A personal injury (or torts) lawyer, Belli represented people who were wrongly hurt by medicines, cars, airplanes, cigarettes, cement trucks, or exploding bottles of Coca-Cola. In the "Close-Up" section of *Life* magazine in October 1954, six months before the Cutter tragedy, Melvin Belli was crowned "the King of Torts." Belli's influence came in part from his insatiable need for media attention—he constantly sought out famous clients. Belli represented Mickey Cohen when he was accused of murdering Las Vegas casino owner Bugsy Siegel; Lenny Bruce, when he was accused of vulgarity in his nightclub act; Evel Knievel, when he wanted permission to jump the Grand Canyon on his motorcycle; Martha Mitchell, when she divorced her husband, Watergate co-conspirator John Mitchell; and Jack Ruby, when he was accused of murdering Lee Harvey Oswald, the man who shot John F. Kennedy.

Belli's need for publicity didn't stop in the courtroom. He played himself in the movies *Wild in the Streets* and *Gimme Shelter;* appeared in episodes of *Hunter, Star Trek,* and *Murder, She Wrote;* and wrote books such as *The Belli Files* and *Melvin Belli: My Life on Trial* (in which he described his five marriages, his naked run down the streets of Berkeley, and his need to inform Parisians of his presence by paging himself at Orly International Airport). After his death an editorial in the *San Francisco Chronicle* stated, "Melvin Belli helped establish the principles of the plaintiff attorney: avarice, immunity to logic, self-aggrandizement, and perfect contempt for the interests of society." Despite his many detractors and flaws, Melvin Belli took on difficult cases, won large claims, and made new law. "He was a very complex guy," remembered Belli's law partner Richard Gerry. "It was extremely interesting to be around him. He was always on the front end of the law; he didn't know when to quit."

In 1956 Josephine and Robert Gottsdanker hired Melvin Belli to represent their daughter Anne, now permanently and severely paralyzed by Cutter's vaccine. (The Gottsdankers' case against Cutter Laboratories also included another child, James "Randy" Phipps, whose left arm and shoulder were paralyzed.) Belli was hesitant: "How could I sue Cutter Laboratories? On the face of it, the Cutter scientists were heroes. Cutter was manufacturing a revolutionary new vaccine that would immunize an entire nation from the deadly effects of infantile paralysis, the disease that crippled President Franklin Delano Roosevelt. Suing Cutter was like suing Florence Nightingale."

Sixty separate civil lawsuits were filed against Cutter Laboratories. Although Eli Lilly, Parke-Davis, and Wyeth were also sued, they settled out of court. Only Cutter chose to take its case to a jury. The case of *Gottsdanker v. Cutter Laboratories* was the first to go to trial, and the verdict determined the outcome of other cases against Cutter. The Gottsdanker verdict also opened a door that affected all pharmaceutical companies for the next fifty years.

Cutter Laboratories was sued on two counts: that it was negligent in producing and testing its vaccine and that it breached a guarantee that its product was what it said it was—namely, an inactivated polio vaccine. "Number one, we claim Cutter was negligent and careless," said Belli, in his opening statement to the jury. "We don't claim that Cutter intended this to happen. We don't claim any criminality. We will show to you that they knew the safety tests were breaking down [and that] they picked up live virus in that vaccine just as it was ready to go out of their doors." Belli said that although there was not a 100 percent guarantee that children would be protected

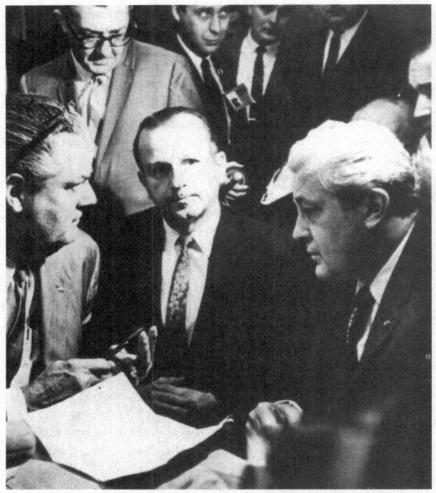

Melvin Belli (right) defending Jack Ruby (center). Ruby was accused of
killing Lee Harvey Oswald, the man who shot John F. Kennedy (reprinted
by permission of SLL/Sterling Lord Literistic, Inc.).

against polio, "there was a 100 percent guarantee, or warranty, that
they would not get polio from the vaccine." Belli was arguing that
if a company prints "inactivated polio vaccine" on the label, it has
by implication guaranteed, or warranted, that its product doesn't
cause polio.

On the morning of Friday, November 22, 1957, two and one-half
years after the Cutter Incident, the case against Cutter Laboratories

began in the Alameda County Courthouse in Oakland, California. In a large, plain room lacking murals, wood paneling, or an imposing dais, Belli linked Cutter Laboratories to his client. He showed that Cutter made a vaccine that was shipped to City Pharmacy in Santa Barbara, California; that William Oliver, Anne Gottsdanker's pediatrician, bought Cutter's vaccine from City Pharmacy; that Anne received Cutter's vaccine by injection into her right upper thigh; that Anne was paralyzed ten days after the injection; that type 1 polio virus was present in Anne's intestines; and that the vaccine that Anne received contained live virulent type 1 polio virus.

Anne sat in the courtroom while her father told the jury what happened during the family's drive back home from Calexico to Santa Barbara, eight days after she had received Cutter's vaccine: "She vomited while she was in the car and said that her head hurt terribly. When we got to El Cajon we stopped off at a medical clinic and saw the physician there, a Dr. Myer. I carried her in. He advised us to get to Santa Barbara as quickly as we could. In the afternoon we saw Dr. Oliver [who] told me that he suspected polio. She began to have considerable pain, not so much in the neck any more, but in the right leg. Then there was pain in the left leg, and we noticed that she couldn't even sit without help."

After Robert Gottsdanker stepped down from the witness chair, Belli turned to Anne and asked her to walk for the jury. Wearing a red sweater to hide her back brace, Anne couldn't hide that both legs were severely paralyzed. "Do I have to show them?" she asked her mother. Using her crutches and brace and under the gentle urgings of her mother and Melvin Belli, Anne haltingly, gamely tried to walk. Later a chilling exchange between Belli and Anne's doctor, Herman Kabat, revealed just how badly Anne had been hurt by Cutter's vaccine:

Belli: And have you any prognosis that you can give the Ladies and Gentlemen of the jury on Anne? What is going to happen to her?

Kabat: She has permanent and complete paralysis of her right [leg].

Belli: Will that get any better?

Kabat: No.

Belli: Will that leg grow equally with the other leg?

Kabat: We don't expect it to, no.

Belli: Any surgery for that?

Kabat: If the shortening is enough it would be necessary to carry out a procedure, a surgical procedure on the left leg to decrease the rate of growth of that leg so that the difference of the [legs] will be less.

Belli: How about the other leg?

Kabat: The other leg has muscles that are severely paralyzed and others that are only partly paralyzed.

Belli: Do you expect to get any improvement of that leg?

Kabat: I wouldn't think so.

Belli: Do you anticipate that there will be any tendon grafts of the [legs]?

Kabat: Just the left.

Belli: Is that tendon transplant a major surgical procedure?

Kabat: Yes.

Belli: How about her back?

Kabat: Her spine shows a definite curvature or scoliosis.

Belli: Will the curve flatten out as the years go on, remain the same, or get worse?

Kabat: The tendency will be for it to get worse.

Belli: Do you have any opinion as to what will have to be done to the spine?

Kabat: Yes, I feel she will need spinal fusion to correct this deformity.

Belli: By spinal fusions, you mean what type of surgery?

Kabat: That would be a grafting of bone on the spine.

Belli had demonstrated to the jury that Cutter's vaccine had paralyzed his client and that Anne's paralysis would be severe, debilitating, and lifelong. Proving that Cutter was negligent would be much harder. Belli called Robert Cutter, president of Cutter Laboratories, to the stand. Cutter walked briskly, confidently forward, but Belli scored points in a brief exchange.

Belli: You didn't intend to sell live virus in your vaccine.

Cutter: How do you define live virus?

Belli: How do you define it? You were making it.

Next, Belli asked that the deposition of his most powerful ally, Jonas Salk, be read in front of the jury. Salk, who gave his deposition to Belli's partner, Lou Ashe, one month before the trial, was furious that Cutter had failed to understand the principles behind his techniques. For the tragedy that occurred in the spring of 1955, Jonas Salk blamed Cutter and Cutter alone.

Ashe: Was the so-called Cutter Incident an industry-wide problem, Doctor?

Salk: No.

Ashe: Did the Cutter Incident disprove the principles and theories which you have enunciated?

Salk: No, [it] did not.

Ashe: Do you have an opinion, Doctor, as to whether [the government requirements of April 12, 1955], set out in connection with your principles, theories, and methods, were sufficient [to make] a vaccine which was safe?

Salk: Yes, the requirements as set forth were [adequate].

Belli called Walter Ward to the stand. Ward was remembered by courtroom observers as "very self-contained, sardonic, slow to speak, intelligent"; he felt that his career had been destroyed and "he was bitter, especially toward Salk, because he believed that [Cutter] followed the instructions in good faith, yet still the vaccine contained live virus. He didn't feel any personal responsibility." Belli confronted Ward with the fact that nine of twenty-seven lots of Cutter's vaccine contained live virus and that although these contaminated lots were further inactivated or destroyed, something was obviously wrong with Cutter's inactivation process.

Belli: You were finding live virus in the vaccine you were manufacturing before you put it out for sale, weren't you?

Ward: We never put out any vaccine for sale in which we found any live virus.

Belli: Isn't it a fair statement that about a third of the vaccines you made were tested positive with live virus?

Ward: That is approximately correct.

Belli: Did you tell the Government the number of lots that you were throwing out in which you got live virus prior to your selling the polio vaccine?

Ward: We were not asked for the information and we did not provide it.

Belli: Didn't you think it was important to show the government that your manufacture was breaking down or that something was going wrong in the way you were producing this vaccine?

Ward: We were all having similar problems.

Belli: Didn't [the inconsistent safety tests] prove to you one of two things: one, that your tests were not accurate, or two, the way you were manufacturing it was wrong?

Ward: Well, I can't answer your question. Something odd or something was going on which scientifically you couldn't explain.

Belli: But you knew that in some tests, one-third of them, you were getting live virus, and something odd was going on, to use your own words, either these tests were not good or your manufacturing was not following the Salk process?

Ward: I just can't answer that question.

Belli: Even at that time, [not] having an answer to that question, you put that vaccine up for sale to the public.

Ward: That's right.

Belli was having trouble proving negligence because he didn't understand the science behind Cutter's mistakes. He had seen virus inactivation graphs showing that Cutter had—more than any other company—completely ignored Salk's concepts. But the science escaped him, so he chose to blame the entire vaccine industry for a cover-up. "No one imagined that Cutter Laboratories would come right out and confess what went wrong," recalled Belli. "I never did discover the whole truth. Cutter Laboratories and the whole goddamn pharmaceutical industry covered up the facts."

Although Ward appeared uncomfortable and evasive on the stand, he had said something that surprised Belli: "We were all having similar problems." Ward put the notion before the jury that Cutter was one of several companies having difficulties. Belli refused to believe this. "It was not called the 'Salk Incident' or the 'Sharp & Dohme Incident' or the 'Lilly Incident' or the 'Wyeth Incident' or the 'Pitman-Moore Incident,' " said Belli. "It was called the 'Cutter Incident' by everyone in and out of the pharmaceutical industry because it was Cutter's vaccine alone which caused the carnage."

Belli countered the testimony of Walter Ward by calling Robert Magoffin to the stand. Magoffin, medical director of the Bureau of Acute Communicable Diseases in California, explained that Cutter's vaccine caused paralysis and that vaccines made by other companies didn't.

> Belli: Did you have an opportunity to compare the vaccinations done by Lilly, Wyeth, Parke-Davis, and other companies making the Salk vaccine?
>
> Magoffin: Yes.
>
> Belli: Will you tell the Ladies and Gentlemen of the jury the conclusions.
>
> Magoffin: In general, we found among individuals who had received Cutter vaccine there was a definitely higher incidence of polio occurring within the first thirty days following inoculation than was observed with the other vaccines used in California.
>
> Belli: That applies to Lilly, Parke-Davis, Wyeth, [and] Pitman-Moore?
>
> Magoffin: Yes, Lilly, Parke-Davis, and a little Pitman-Moore were the only other vaccines used in California.

Belli had almost gotten what he wanted. Magoffin said that vaccines made by Lilly, Parke-Davis, and Pitman-Moore didn't cause paralysis; he had omitted Wyeth because Wyeth hadn't distributed its vaccine in California. Cutter's defense team noticed the omission. Belli called Walter Ward back to the stand.

> Belli: You do know there is a white paper, or whatever it is called, put out by the government, showing that Lilly had absolutely no live virus in the way they manufactured the Salk vaccine in over 2,000,000 injections?

> Ward: I know there is a white paper, and I also know that this white paper shows [other] manufacturers also had [problems].

The "white paper" to which Belli referred stated that the incidence of paralysis following immunization with vaccines made by Lilly, Parke-Davis, and Pitman-Moore was not statistically different from the incidence of natural polio. But Ward had seen the report and knew that it also showed that all five manufacturers had had difficulties inactivating polio virus. Cutter's lawyers pounced on the opening. The defense team was led by Wallace Sedgwick, a "charming, engaging, confident" man and Belli's opposite in style and character. Sedgwick called Howard Shaughnessy (the director of the laboratory of the Illinois Health Department) to the stand. As a polio expert, Shaughnessy had served on an advisory committee to the federal government following the Cutter tragedy, and he had seen the virus inactivation data from all companies, including Wyeth, during committee meetings. He was one of the few people in the courtroom who knew about the recalled lot of Wyeth's vaccine.

> Sedgwick: Was any of the Wyeth vaccine recalled?

> Shaughnessy: Yes. That was known to me personally, one lot.

> Sedgwick: Can you tell us the reason it was withdrawn?

> Shaughnessy: Because 11 cases of polio were found to be associated with the use of that material.

Surprised by the contention that Wyeth might have made a vaccine that paralyzed children, Belli began to cross-examine Shaughnessy. Belli was about to commit a fundamental error of cross-examination: he would ask a question to which he didn't know the answer.

Belli: Is it your testimony that the vaccine of the other manufacturers wasn't clear and held to be free from live virus; is that your testimony?

Shaughnessy: As of that time, live virus had not been found in material which had been sold by other manufacturers, or by Cutter.

Belli: Or by Cutter?

Shaughnessy: Or by Cutter, as of May 5 and 6.

Belli: Why was Cutter withdrawn?

Shaughnessy: On the basis of epidemiologic evidence entirely as of that date.

Belli: But no vaccine of any other manufacturer was withdrawn on the basis of any other epidemiological certainty?

Shaughnessy: Yes, one lot.

Belli: Was it, or wasn't it?

Shaughnessy: It was.

Belli hesitated, uncertain how to proceed. He hadn't known that Wyeth's vaccine had been recalled. "I understand him to say 'Yes,'" the judge said, urging Belli to continue. Shaughnessy repeated his answer.

Shaughnessy: One lot of Wyeth was withdrawn.

Belli: And that was subsequently cleared?

Shaughnessy: I know of no evidence of that.

In his closing argument, Belli did his best to minimize the testimony that Wyeth had made a vaccine that paralyzed children and that all five companies had had problems inactivating polio virus. He knew that if the problem of virus inactivation was perceived as industry-wide, it would be hard for the jury to find Cutter negligent. "We thought and thought a long time on this," Belli told the jury. "We can find no responsibility on Dr. Salk. Similarly, we find no responsibility on the National Foundation, and no responsibility whatsoever on the part of the government. . . . There can be no blame attached to these

other people and once you start going through the transcript, I think
you will see, Ladies and Gentlemen, why the fault of this unique
incident, not being industry wide, was Cutter's and Cutter's alone."

Belli concluded that if medicine was a process of evolution, Anne
Gottsdanker shouldn't have to pay for the process. "There is, as a
matter of law [the notion] that you cannot assume a risk in a case
like this. Maybe only a few got [paralyzed]. Maybe science advanced.
Maybe science must advance over the bodies of the young and old and
the twisted and the lame, [but] there is no doubt in my mind—and
there should be none in yours—that the process could and should be
perfect."

Cutter's defense team wanted to show that Cutter had followed government regulations; that Salk's straight-line theory of virus inactivation was difficult to reproduce on a commercial scale; and that the
process of making a polio vaccine was not far enough advanced to
allow any company to make a vaccine that could be declared, with
confidence, free from live virus. (It also wanted to tell the jury that
Cutter had vaccinated the children of 450 employees, but Belli successfully excluded this testimony in pre-trial hearings.)

Wallace Sedgwick was forty-nine years old, with thinning hair and
a ruddy complexion. A native of Mexico City, Sedgwick had received
his law degree from Southwestern University in Los Angeles, California, and as a recognized expert in insurance law, he frequently lec-
tured to professional organizations. He was hired by Cutter's insurance company. Sedgwick was an excellent trial lawyer. James Gault,
Sedgwick's law partner, remembered:

> When I first came with the firm, I was consumed by work and I couldn't smile
> and I couldn't laugh and I was just slaving away. We had a maintenance man, a
> janitor, who would come by at about six or seven o'clock in the evening and
> empty the wastepaper baskets, dust off the desks, and clean out the ashtrays. He
> was a really glum guy and he never smiled. My office was very close to Sedg-
> wick's, and he would come to my office first, and I'd want him to get in and out
> fast because I had all of this work to do. I noticed that he would then go into
> Sedgwick's office and the door would close and he would be in there for the
> longest time and I couldn't figure out what was going on. I later found out that
> every time he went in, Sedgwick engaged him in conversation and wanted to
> know what was going on in his life and how things were. The janitor would walk

out of the office just beaming, shoulders back, head up, smiling, humming a
tune. Sedgwick just got him turned around. He'd go in depressed and came out a
new man. Sedgwick was really interested in people.

Wallace Sedgwick began his defense of Cutter Laboratories by
calling William Workman (director of the Laboratory of Biologics
Control) to the stand. Sedgwick was determined to show the jury that
in the spring of 1955 government requirements were inadequate to
ensure a safe polio vaccine and that all companies were having trouble
consistently and completely inactivating polio virus.

Sedgwick: Now, would you tell us what you know about the experience of
manufacturers in general . . . as to whether or not they had what we call failure of
a lot, because the test showed the presence of live virus? Did it occur?

Workman: Yes, it did.

Sedgwick: Will you describe the frequency or irregularity or whatever it may
have been in that experience in general terms?

Workman: Of the 809 lots tabulated for all [vaccine manufacturers], 11 percent
were positive.

Sedgwick: In your opinion were the [government] requirements in effect on
April 12, 1955, adequate to assure the consistent safety or absence of live virus of
a vaccine produced in accordance with such requirements?

Workman: My opinion is . . . that they were not. However, the [government]
requirements of April 12, 1955, did represent the best knowledge and experience
available as of that date.

Sedgwick: In your opinion, Dr. Workman, did the evidence and information
available to you show that Cutter Laboratories did follow the methods and
procedures set out by the [government] requirements?

Workman: I was not able to obtain any evidence that the Cutter Laboratories
had failed to comply with the government regulations or requirements then in
effect.

Next, Sedgwick called Wendell Stanley to the stand. Sedgwick
asked Stanley to describe his credentials as a chemist and virologist and
then asked if he had ever received a Nobel Prize. Stanley, after a dramatic pause, answered, "Yes." Stanley laid the blame for the Cutter

tragedy at the feet of Jonas Salk and his straight-line theory of inactivation. He believed that asking companies to completely inactivate polio
virus using Salk's method was asking them to do the impossible.

> Sedgwick: Is the reaction of formaldehyde on polio virus a multiple or a [straight-
> line] reaction?

> Stanley: I would say from the standpoint of theory, you would not expect the
> interaction between formaldehyde and polio virus . . . to be a [straight-line]
> reaction.

> Sedgwick: What is your opinion as to whether or not the [government] require-
> ments were adequate or inadequate as of April 12, 1955?

> Stanley: In the light of subsequent knowledge, they were grossly inadequate.

Belli remembered the fanfare surrounding Wendell Stanley's appearance. "Cutter didn't tell us who their defense witnesses would be.
In those days, the defense didn't have to reveal this information before
trial. But after we'd finished putting on our case, I noticed a lot of
flashbulbs popping in the corridor and learned that Wally Sedgwick
was out there introducing one of his star witnesses to the press. It was
Dr. Wendell Stanley, a Nobel Prize winner. It took Sedgwick half a day
to run through all of Dr. Stanley's degrees and honors and associations
and another half day for Dr. Stanley to snow the jury with his tales
about viruses, which, he said, are 'almost like crystals.' You don't
know, he told the jury, whether the crystals are living or dead, they can
procreate, they have 'a personality.' Jesus the jury was spellbound."

During preparation for the trial, Sedgwick, realizing that federal
requirements for production of polio vaccine were inadequate, asked
Robert Cutter whether he wanted to sue the government to deflect the
blame. The recommendation to put the government on trial was made
by Sedgwick's co-counsel, Scott Conley. "I felt at the time and actually
recommended to our law firm that a lawsuit be filed against the federal
government and Oveta Culp Hobby," Conley recalled. "I felt that that
would . . . be a dramatic counterpoint and would give the jury someone
else to look at as the responsible party. There was also some thought to
[suing] Dr. Salk, but Dr. Salk was such a cult figure, he was such a hero
at that time, that I thought it would be counterproductive. I wish

we had done it." After much consideration and largely because Cutter Laboratories—like all pharmaceutical companies—depended on the federal government to license its products, Robert Cutter rejected the strategy.

Next, Sedgwick called Karl Habel to the stand. Habel had been sent by William Workman to Berkeley to investigate Cutter Laboratories immediately after the first signs of the tragedy.

> Sedgwick: Could you tell us what your conclusions were in the reports that you made?

> Habel: My conclusion was that we found no evidence of negligence or purposeful evasion of the [government] requirements. My own conclusions at the time were that the inactivation procedure and in general the manufacture of the polio vaccine was not at the stage where it could be called a standard process. And it seemed apparent that the safety tests, as performed at that time, even when carried out correctly and adequately, could not be sure of completely eliminating the possibility that small amounts of live virus might be in the final product. This applied not only to Cutter, but to the procedures themselves.

Belli had been surprised to hear that all manufacturers had had trouble consistently inactivating polio virus and that Wyeth had made one lot of vaccine that was withdrawn from the market. During the testimony of Edwin Lennette, the director of the Virus Laboratory for the State of California, Belli would be surprised one more time. Lennette was about to testify that Cutter's was not an isolated incident.

> Lennette: What we are discussing here today is not without precedent. This sort of thing we are discussing [happened] with the Venezuelan equine encephalitis [vaccine]. Here we have a virus that was, by all laboratory tests one could devise, inactivated, and yet produced human infections when administered to people.

> Belli: That is the. . . .

> Lennette: Venezeulan equine encephalitis [vaccine].

Belli quickly changed the subject—but the damage was done. Venezuelan equine encephalitis was a virus that was first found to infect horses in Colombia, South America, in the 1930s. It soon became clear that the virus infected other species, including humans, and caused disease in many countries. Injected into the bloodstream by the bite of a mosquito, the virus caused swelling of the brain (encephalitis) and inflammation of the lining of the brain and spinal cord (meningitis). Although the disease was usually mild, it was occasionally severe—causing permanent brain damage—and sometimes fatal. The army was interested in a vaccine to prevent Venezuelan equine encephalitis because military personnel and laboratory researchers occasionally got the disease. In 1954 the army made a vaccine by inactivating Venezuelan equine encephalitis virus with formaldehyde, a process virtually identical to that used by Jonas Salk to inactivate polio virus. The vaccine was given to 327 people.

On February 2, 1954, one year before the Cutter tragedy, a forty-year-old fireman from Maryland was admitted to the hospital with fever, chills, and severe headaches. Fearing meningitis, doctors performed a spinal tap. Normally people have no white blood cells (cells that the body uses to fight infection) in their spinal fluid, but the fireman had 5,750 of them. During the next several months thirteen more men were admitted to the hospital. All had fever, headaches, meningitis, and encephalitis; all had recently received the "inactivated" Venezuelan equine encephalitis vaccine; and all were found to have live, potentially deadly Venezuelan equine encephalitis virus in their blood. Like Cutter's polio vaccine, scientists had made Venezuelan equine encephalitis vaccine by growing the virus in animal cells, filtering the virus-cell mixture before inactivation, completely inactivating the virus with formaldehyde, and testing the vaccine in animals to make sure that it didn't contain live virus. And like Cutter's polio vaccine, the Venezuelan equine encephalitis vaccine inadvertently caused the disease that it was intended to prevent. The jury was learning that medicine was apparently an inescapable process of trial and error. When Sedgwick cross-examined Lennette, he came back to the subject of Venezuelan equine encephalitis vaccine.

Sedgwick: You were asked a question about this Venezuelan equine encephalitis [vaccine] and you started to explain what it was. Will you tell us what it is, first?

Lennette: This was the reference, I believe, to the fact that virus may be inactivated and still cause difficulties in the human. When the vaccine was used in humans to immunize them, out of some 300 [people], there were 14 cases of Venezuelan equine encephalitis, clinical cases. Some 200 guinea pigs were inoculated, some 6,000 mice and no one ever got the virus out; the point being here that all the safety tests passed without deviation showing the virus to be safe and inactivated or dead, and in the final host, man, it came to life. *The final criterion of whether a thing is inactivated for man is to put it into man, is what it amounts to.*

The experience with the Venezuelan equine encephalitis vaccine was exactly analogous to the inactivated polio vaccine: evidence that inactivation methods were unreliable and that safety tests were inadequate was found only after immunizing people.

On January 14, 1958, fifty-two days after the beginning of the trial, Wallace Sedgwick gave his closing arguments. The rigors of a long trial had taken a toll. Too ill to stand, his voice broken by laryngitis, Sedgwick sat on a chair in front of the jury.

"We are charged first and foremost . . . as being negligent and careless in the manufacture of the vaccine so that it caused the injuries to these plaintiffs. We are also charged with having breached some warranties. First, negligence, briefly, is the doing of something that, in the exercise of ordinary care, you should not do; or failure to do something that, in the exercise of ordinary care, you should do." Sedgwick argued that Cutter wasn't negligent because manufacturing protocols and safety tests weren't far enough advanced in the spring of 1955 to assure the absence of live virus—only knowledge gained from the Cutter tragedy had allowed such assurances. "You don't criticize the Wright Brothers because the first airplane did not act like today's airliners. Nor can you compare an early model T Ford with today's high-powered cars. But you don't criticize the people that worked with those devices in the early days. . . . And isn't that what happened here? There have been developments and there have been improvements. People are human. We don't know everything when we start out on any given job." Sedgwick continued: "The second charge is that we breached a warranty. Now, Ladies and Gentlemen, you won't hear the term 'absolute liability' from His Honor, I am certain because that is not the law and it does not apply here. . . . What do we warrant? . . . If you buy a lawnmower, it is supposed to cut the lawn. That is the implied warranty. But you don't warrant something that is not yet known. You don't warrant knowledge of scientific advances that are not yet made."

Before the jury went to the jury room, it heard instructions from the judge, Thomas J. Ledwich. A small man with a full head of gray-white hair, Ledwich was described by both plaintiff and defense attorneys as stubborn, willful, and unimpressive. Ledwich didn't make up his own instructions. Rather, he sorted through forty-nine proposed instructions by Sedgwick and sixty-two by Belli. He decided which ones to accept and which ones to reject. His choices directed the verdict.

Sedgwick didn't want Cutter to be left holding the bag for a process that wasn't perfected. He asked the judge to say, "In determining whether the vaccine injected into plaintiffs was reasonably fit for its intended purpose, you must remember that the issue is whether the vaccine was reasonably fit *as of the time it was injected* into the plaintiffs, and not whether it was reasonably fit according to present day standards." Also, during his closing argument, Wallace Sedgwick had said, "You won't hear the term 'absolute liability' from His Honor." Sedgwick asked the judge to back him up by saying, "The implied warranty that an article is reasonably fit for the purpose intended does not mean that the seller warrants *the absolute safety* of the article." Ledwich denied both of Sedgwick's requested instructions.

Belli fared much better. He asked for and received two critical instructions that supported his case. Belli asked the judge to undermine Cutter's contention that compliance with government regulations was good enough. Ledwich agreed and said to the jury, "Defendant Cutter Laboratories contends that it complied with the minimum requirements of the United States Department of Health, Education, and Welfare for the production of polio vaccine. In this regard, I instruct you that *compliance with those requirements will not relieve the defendant of liability.*" Belli also asked for and received an instruction that tied the hands of the jury and opened the door for a revolution in product liability law: he asked that the judge make Cutter liable for a process that was not, at the time of manufacture, adequate to ensure absolute safety.

At 10:00 A.M. on Thursday, January 16, 1958, Thomas Ledwich addressed the jury: "Upon all questions of law it is your duty to be guided by the instructions of the Court and to accept the law as given to you by the Court, whether you agree with it or not." For one hour and forty-five minutes, Ledwich defined terms such as "negligence," "implied warranty," "express warranty," "merchantability," and "fitness for purpose." His final words to the jury sealed Cutter's fate: "If you find that the vaccine of defendant Cutter Laboratories did in fact contain infectious amounts of live polio virus, and that the injection of vaccine into the minor plaintiffs [caused] polio, [then] I instruct you that the defendant Cutter Laboratories breached an implied warranty." Ledwich was saying that if Cutter's vaccine had paralyzed Anne Gottsdanker, then the jury had no choice but to find Cutter guilty.

On January 16, 1958, at 11:44 A.M., twelve jurors, accompanied by the bailiff, walked to the jury room and began their deliberations. Later that day the jurors asked to review several pieces of evidence. They wanted to see the *Technical Report* that described how all five pharmaceutical companies had had trouble inactivating polio virus. They wanted to see government requirements for production of polio vaccine at the time of the Cutter tragedy. They wanted to see the World Health Organization report of the meeting in Geneva in 1957 that showed, two years after the Cutter tragedy, that the type of filter manufacturers picked was critical to making a safe vaccine. Clearly the jurors were having trouble buying into Belli's contention that Cutter had been negligent. But they also asked for one piece of information that angered Ledwich. Uncomfortable with the judge's instructions, they wanted to see how "implied warranty" was defined in law books.

Judge: Now, the other question you asked was whether you could have the Civil Code in the jury room relating to implied warranty; and, if not, you request that I re-read the law to you. It is not customary to send law books or excerpts from the law to the jury room, especially not law books. Therefore, I will re-read to you the definition of implied warranty: "Where the buyer, expressly or by implication, makes known to the seller the particular purpose for which goods are required, and it appears that the buyer relies on the seller's skill or judgment . . . there is an implied warranty that the goods shall be reasonably fit for such purpose."

After twelve hours and forty minutes of deliberation, on Friday, January 17, 1958, the jury, led by the foreman, James Watters, returned to the courtroom with a verdict. Fred Cutter, Robert Cutter's younger brother, was sitting in the courtroom when the bailiff handed the verdict to the judge. He remembered the confusion that followed:

"The judge read and reread the verdict to himself and very evidently puzzled over it as the court waited. Finally, after several minutes of deliberation, he invited counsel for both sides into his chambers. More time elapsed with the court buzzing, but still no inkling as to the verdict." Ledwich silently read what the jury had written: "We, the jury find in favor of Anne Elizabeth Gottsdanker and against Cutter Laboratories and assess damages in the sum of $125,000." Next to the word "Verdict" was written in pencil the phrase "as explained on accompanying sheets." The jurors had difficulty saying that a company was liable when they didn't feel that the company was negligent; they felt compelled to explain what they had done:

> Your Honor,
>
> On the assumption that the attached forms of verdict were prepared for us merely as a convenience, we submit that it is our right and duty to expand upon it briefly. We feel that the Court would wish to know the full extent of the verdict agreed upon.
>
> The jury took as first consideration the matter of negligence, and from a preponderance of the evidence concluded that the defendant, Cutter Laboratories, was not negligent either directly or by inference in producing and selling polio vaccine under conditions prevailing at the time of the Cutter incident.
>
> With regard to the law of warranty, however, we feel that we have no alternative but to conclude that Cutter Laboratories [brought] to market a lot of vaccine which when given to plaintiffs caused them to come down with polio, this resulting in a breach of warranty. For this cause alone we find in favor of the plaintiffs.
>
> Signed, James T. Watters (Foreman)

Ledwich had been on the bench for twenty-two years. He had been handed verdicts of "liable" and "not liable, " but he had never been handed a verdict of "liable with an explanation." When he saw the sheet that accompanied the verdicts, he hesitated before allowing the bailiff to read them aloud.

> Judge: The jury will remain seated a minute. Well, I will have the Clerk read the verdicts of the jury and then—the jury will remain seated a few minutes. I want to take a matter up in chambers with counsel before proceeding with the verdicts.

Before Ledwich read the verdict to the lawyers, he brought Belli, Sedgwick, the court reporter (Lillian Cohn), and the deputy county clerk (Frank Veit) into his chambers.

Judge: Without saying anything further about the verdicts, the verdict in each case is headed "Verdict of the Jury" in the form it was presented to the jury; then there is written opposite those words, in lead pencil, "As explained on accompanying sheets," and then there is an explanation of what they want to go with their verdict. I am of the opinion offhand that the only thing their verdict is is what they have signed here as the verdict without reference to these sheets, but I don't know. I have never run into a situation like this before.

Sedgwick: I think if they refer to something, we ought to have a record of it. It is part of it.

Judge: Possibly so. I don't know. Have you ever run into this, Mr. Belli?

Belli: I will try to think.

Judge: Have you ever run into it, Frank? Frank used to be with Judge Gray, and was my Clerk for seven years. Have you ever run into anything attached to a verdict, Frank?

Veit: Way back. I just can't recall all the details, but do you want to know what was done?

Judge: Yes.

Veit: The Judge . . . would permit the verdict to stand, but only that which the Jury Foreman put his signature to would count. It wasn't exactly like this one.

Sedgwick: Wouldn't it be easier to read it into the record so that we know what we are talking about?

Belli: I stipulate to that.

Sedgwick: My suggestion is that it is impossible for Mr. Belli or me to discuss with the Court, and intelligently, what the problem is until we know. Can we informally read into the record everything that is on the sheets in your hand and on the verdict and then will we know what is necessary.

Belli: I stipulate it be read. However, I think the verdict is the verdict signed.

The group walked back to the courtroom; Ledwich handed the verdicts to the bailiff; and after they were read, said, "Mr. Clerk, you will read the verdicts to the jury and ascertain if they are their true and correct verdicts." On the charge of negligence, the vote was 10-2 in favor of Cutter. On the charge of implied warranty, the vote was 11-1 against Cutter. (In civil cases such as *Gottsdanker v. Cutter Laboratories,* the jury does not have to be unanimous to reach a decision; only a majority of votes is required.)

Ledwich decided later that the accompanying sheet did not have separate legal standing. His decision was based on a code of civil procedure that stated, "An attempt by the jury to decide upon what theory of law it renders its verdict is beyond its function in determining a general verdict for or against the defendant." But the defense team was impressed with the jury's clarity and thoughtfulness: "They understood the issues perfectly," said James Gault. "The accompanying sheet was an articulate statement of their position. It was beautifully written."

Both sides claimed victory.

Publicly Belli boasted that the decision "was easily the most spectacular development in modern tort law—the most potent new weapon aimed at making business safeguard consumers. I had started out to prove 'warranty.' The court went beyond my contentions and held on 'absolute liability' or 'liability without fault.'" Privately, Belli was disappointed with the outcome. Three days after the trial he wrote a letter to Jonas Salk—and included an autographed copy of a book about himself. "I was disappointed in the Cutter verdict," said Belli, "both in the amount and the imposition and basis of liability. The jury found . . . not only that Cutter was not negligent, they by implication found that Cutter's 'team of scientists' were telling the truth. I can begin to appreciate something of what you went through when I come up against these 'scientists.' I am sorry we didn't 'let them have it' a little bit stronger in the deposition. They not only deserved it but were asking for it. However, had we not had your deposition at all, I am sure they would have gotten away with a defense verdict and not only slandered you and the program but proved that the children didn't get polio at all—it was just our imagination!" Salk replied: "I read of the verdict with considerable interest and realize the vagaries of juries, and the distinction between seeking truth and justice. They should be, but not always are, one and the same."

Several weeks after the verdict Robert Cutter wrote a letter to Cutter's shareholders and customers: "The first polio vaccine suit has just recently been completed. . . . The jury was remarkable. They listened to technical evidence for over six weeks. They refused to be confused. They felt that the interpretation of the law, which made it mandatory for them to find for the plaintiffs on implied warranty, was so harsh that they insisted that the following statement be made part of the verdict: 'Cutter Laboratories was not negligent, either directly or by inference.' I can't tell you how much I appreciate the substantial support we have had from you in the medical and allied professions throughout this entire ordeal. Even in the darkest day when no one knew what had happened, you never lost confidence. May you *never* have to make excuses for us."

Several jurors said they regarded the verdict as "extremely harsh." Anita Steiner said, "We felt obligated to follow the law, whether we agreed with it or not"; Jennie Tennant complained that the verdict was "directed" by the judge; and James Watters, a credit analyst for Wells Fargo Bank and the jury's foreman said, "We were appalled by the simplicity of the jury forms given us to register our verdict." The criticism angered Ledwich: "It boiled down to this—did the children get polio from the vaccine or didn't they? You can call it a directed verdict."

As a consequence of Melvin Belli's proposed instructions and under the strong hand of Judge Thomas J. Ledwich, a jury of twelve men and women in Oakland, California, had reluctantly opened Pandora's Box.

Cigars, Parasites, and Human Toes

What the legal process invented in the 1960s came to be called strict liability. . . . A more accurate name would have been more liability. All that the new system could promise, and all it ever delivered, was more lawyers and more litigation.
—Peter Huber

THE JURY HAD FOUND THAT CUTTER LABORATO-ries was not negligent in the production of polio vaccine, but Cutter was still financially responsible (liable) for harm caused by its product. Liability without negligence (fault) was born. The Gottsdanker verdict meant that if pharmaceutical companies made a product according to industry standards, using the best science that was available, and found months or years after its sale that it caused harm—a harm not predictable—they were liable for the damage. Melvin Belli understood that the Gottsdanker decision was a blueprint for a revolution. "It is going to change the face of the legal map," said Belli. "We'll have thousands of [the new law] printed [and] ship them to law libraries and law offices and courts all over the world."

The court decision that held pharmaceutical companies responsible for their products—even when they weren't negligent in the design or manufacture of those products—was the last in a series of important decisions, all of which were made in the United States. But the regulation of products began in England in the thirteenth century, under the reign of King John. In medieval England, if vendors sold spoiled meat, stale bread, or bad beer, they were sent to the pillory. Offenders included the following:

> Sprowston men [who] knowingly [bought] measly pigs, and [sold] the sausages and puddings, unfit for human bodies, in the Norwich market.
>
> John Geggard, [who] bought a dead cow at Earlham and sold it for good sound meat in Norwich.

John Janne [who] bought from Alan de Catton eight drowned sheep and sold them for good meat.

Regulation of the marketplace ensured a fair measure and a minimum standard of quality. But unlike Anne Gottsdanker, a person harmed by a product in thirteenth-century England wasn't compensated for his or her loss; rather, the seller was fined or publicly embarrassed. Compensation for damages came later.

In 1929 an eighteen-year-old boy named George Hawkins inadvertently burned the palm of his right hand with an electrical wire. In an effort to remove "a considerable quantity of scar tissue," he contracted the services of Edward McGee, a local physician. McGee said that he would replace the scar with a skin graft taken from Hawkins's chest and that Hawkins could expect "a one hundred percent perfect hand." The surgery failed. Instead of having a normal hand without a scar, Hawkins had a mangled hand with small tufts of hair growing out of it. Hawkins sued McGee and won.

George Hawkins's lawsuit against Edward McGee featured three legal tenets: there was a direct interaction between the two men (*contract*); a statement by the doctor that he could remove the scar (*express warranty*); and the promise of a functional hand without a scar replaced by the reality of a dysfunctional hand with chest hair growing out of it (*negligence*). Between the early 1800s and the mid-1950s, each of these requirements (contract, express warranty, and negligence) became unnecessary for a plaintiff to successfully claim damages.

The first requirement to fall was express warranty. In 1829 in England a certain Mr. Jones was interested in buying copper sheathing to protect the bottom of his boat. He was introduced by a mutual friend to Mr. Bright, who said, "Your friend may depend on it, we will supply him well." Jones purchased one thousand sheets of copper from Bright for £300 and set off on his boat, the *Isabella,* for a trip from England to Sierra Leone. But instead of the copper lasting four to five years, it was "greatly corroded and of little or no value" in four months. Jones sued Bright for his loss. Although Jones and Bright had a direct interaction (contract), the contract never expressly stated that the copper would last for several years (express warranty). The judge ruled that although the length of time that the copper would last was not stated, it was implied (implied warranty): "When an article is sold for a particular purpose, a warranty is implied that it is fit for that purpose."

From Roman times to the Industrial Revolution people made products in their homes, so there was little need to protect the buyer. Buyers were simply warned to be careful (*caveat emptor,* or "buyer beware"). With the Industrial Revolution, it became clear that a buyer was unlikely to have the expertise to understand how companies or individuals made certain products, like copper; so the law was extended to include implied warranty. Still, a buyer could sue only if there had been a direct interaction (contract) with the seller.

The next requirement to fall was contract. On July 21, 1936, Alvina Klein sent her husband, Herbert, into the Happy Daze Buffet to buy a ham and cheese sandwich. Herbert bought the sandwich, walked back to the car, and handed it to his wife, who took a bite and swallowed it. Alvina noted a "peculiar taste" and immediately examined the sandwich to find that it was "crawling with worms or maggots." She became ill and vomited. During the next six months Alvina Klein withdrew to a sanitarium with "a marked nervousness and obsession against food." She sued the maker of the sandwich, the Duchess Sandwich Company. Although Alvina didn't have a contract with Duchess—and wasn't even the person who bought the sandwich—the judge ruled that "the remedies of an injured consumer of unwholesome food should not be made to rest solely on . . . contract."

The ruling in the case of Alvina Klein and her worm-infested ham and cheese sandwich included two important components. First, a contract between a buyer and seller was no longer required to claim damages. Second, the buyer didn't have to prove that the seller was negligent if negligence was obvious. Negligence could be implied from a rule of evidence called *res ipsa loquitor* (the thing speaks for itself). Several other cases had been decided on this standard of evidence.

In 1915 Mrs. Lou Boyd of Nashville, Tennessee, bought a bottle of Coca-Cola for its "invigorating effects." She opened the sealed top, poured it into a glass, drank it, and "immediately became intensely nauseated." Mrs. Boyd examined the bottle and found a cigar stub about two inches long that "had apparently been in the liquid for some time." She sued the Coca-Cola Bottling Company and won. In 1918 Bryson Pillars of Jackson, Mississippi, bought a pouch of Brown Mule Chewing Tobacco made by the R. J. Reynolds Tobacco Company. Pillars consumed the first few plugs of tobacco without difficulty, but later, feeling "sicker and sicker," his teeth struck "something hard." He examined the pouch and found a "human toe with flesh and nail intact." A physician said that Pillars's illness was caused by poison generated by the rotting toe. Judges on appeal ruled against R. J. Reynolds, stating, "We can imagine no reason why, with ordinary care, human toes could not be left out of chewing tobacco; and if toes are found in chewing tobacco, it seems to us that somebody has been very careless." In October 1938 Yolanda Vaccarezza purchased four salamis from the G. B. Celli Company, owned by Peter and Raphael Sanguinetti. Several weeks after eating the salami—made from "uncooked beef, pork, spices, and salt"—Yolanda and her two sons developed fever, muscle pain, swelling around the eyes, and pain on moving the eyes. A biopsy of Yolanda's muscles showed that she had trichinosis, a disease caused by eating meat infested with the larvae of a pork tapeworm. The Vaccarezzas sued the Sanguinettis for negligence and won.

The importance of contract is best shown in the story of the Massengill Company of Bristol, Tennessee, which produced antibiotics. One year after Alvina Klein bit into her worm-infested sandwich, the courts held Massengill liable even though the company didn't have a direct contract with consumers of its product. In 1937 the first antibiotic, sulfanilamide, was sold to the public. Because sulfanilamide was synthesized in 1908, it was not protected by patents, and several pharmaceutical companies (including Squibb, Merck, Winthrop, Eli Lilly, and Parke-Davis) made it; companies sold sulfanilamide in the form of a capsule or tablet. Massengill decided to make the drug more palatable for children by suspending it in liquid. Unfortunately, sulfanilamide wasn't soluble in liquids typically used by pharmaceutical companies, such as water and alcohol. But the chief chemist for Massengill, Harold Watkins, found that sulfanilamide was soluble in diethylene glycol, an industrial solvent. The final preparation—called "Elixir Sulfanilamide" —contained 72 percent diethylene glycol, 10 percent sulfanilamide, 16 percent water, and small amounts of raspberry extract, saccharin, caramel, and amaranth, which gave the elixir a deep, reddish-purple color. Massengill tested the elixir for fragrance, flavor, and appearance but—because it was not required to—never for safety. Although diethylene glycol had never been tested in people, it had been tested in animals. Ten months earlier Massengill had found that rats developed kidney failure and died after drinking a 3 percent solution of diethylene glycol; although animal studies did not always predict problems in humans, Massengill's product contained a concentration of diethylene glycol that was 24 times greater than that tested in rats.

In September 1937, 240 gallons of Elixir Sulfanilamide were distributed across the United States, and during the next four weeks 353 people drank it. Soon after ingestion, people developed heartburn, nausea, cramps, dizziness, vomiting, diarrhea, difficulty breathing, kidney failure (like the rats), and coma; 105 died, 34 of whom were young children. A representative of the Food and Drug Administration described Massengill's drug development strategy as throwing "drugs together and if they don't explode placing them on sale." After the tragedy the president of Massengill said, "My chemists and I deeply regret the fatal results, but there was no error in the manufacture of the product. We have been supplying legitimate professional demand and not once could have foreseen the unlooked for results. I do not feel that there was any responsibility on our part." The company wasn't obligated much beyond its remorse; it paid a fine of $26,100 for "misbranding." Howard Watkins expressed his remorse by killing himself. As a consequence of the Massengill disaster, Congress passed the Food, Drug, and Cosmetic Act in 1938. The act required companies to test their products for safety before selling them.

The last to fall was negligence. In 1944 Gladys Escola, a waitress in Madera, California, was putting bottles of Coca-Cola into a refrigerator when one of them exploded. The bottle broke into "two jagged pieces, and inflicted a deep five-inch cut, severing blood vessels, nerves, and muscles of the thumb and palm." Gladys Escola's hand was damaged irreparably. Her lawyer, Melvin Belli, claimed that although negligence on the part of the Coca-Cola Bottling Company was not obvious—and, unlike the food, beverage, and tobacco cases, could not be assumed—he did not have to prove negligence to win damages. Belli wanted to make companies financially responsible for harm caused by their products even if they weren't negligent in producing them. Justice Roger Traynor agreed: "I believe the manufacturer's negligence should no longer be singled out as the basis of plaintiff's right to recover in cases like the present one. In my opinion, it should now be recognized that a manufacturer incurs an *absolute liability* when an article that he has placed on the market . . . proves to have a defect that causes injury to human beings." Belli understood the importance of the Escola decision: thirty years later he said, "If there is one legal decision upon which Ralph Nader built, this was it."

The doors had been knocked down for foods, beverages, and tobacco. Plaintiffs no longer had to have a contract with or a promise from a seller or prove negligence by a seller to claim damages. It took another ten years—with *Gottsdanker v. Cutter Laboratories*—to extend the standard of liability without fault to pharmaceutical companies. Because negligence was no longer required, judges and juries focused their attention on the product—and away from the company. The law had shifted from buyer beware (*caveat emptor*) to seller beware (*caveat vendor*).

Wallace Sedgwick's only chance to save pharmaceutical companies from liability without fault was to appeal the Gottsdanker verdict to the District Court of Appeals of the State of California. His appeal consisted of several arguments. Sedgwick claimed that it was much easier to find cigars in bottles of Coca-Cola and human toes in pouches of chewing tobacco than it was to find live polio virus in a polio vaccine: "Adulterants, spoilage, or deleterious substances in food are either visible or easily tested by relatively simple procedures, and toxic or infectious substances in food can be avoided with reasonable certainty. By contrast, pharmaceutical products and biologic products are groping redemptions from the unknown." Polio virus couldn't be reliably found in polio vaccine in April 1955 because fail-safe tests to detect polio virus weren't developed until later. Sedgwick claimed that the result of the verdict made Cutter "the guarantor of the scientifically unknowable, the warrantor of the future." To support his contention, he cited a civil code that stated, "No man shall be responsible for that which no man can control," and a ruling in a Maine court in 1912 that stated, "Neither law nor reason requires impossibilities."

Sedgwick claimed that strict liability standards for foods included only foreign substances that shouldn't be there—for example, cigars, parasites, and toes. He argued that those standards shouldn't apply to substances that were part of the original product: "Under the standards of producing foodstuffs at the time, companies were not held liable if there was a chicken bone in chicken pie [or] small oyster shells present in canned oysters." Sedgwick reasoned that small quantities of live polio virus were present in an inactivated polio vaccine for the same reason that small quantities of chicken bones or oyster shells were present in chicken pies or cans of oysters: it was the standard of the industry. In support of his argument, Sedgwick reminded the court of the subtle warning of the National Foundation during the field trial of Salk's vaccine in 1954: "The possibility of infectious activity remaining in any vaccine . . . has been reduced to a point below which it cannot be measured by practicable laboratory procedures."

Sedgwick claimed that even if there had been a contract between Anne Gottsdanker and Cutter Laboratories, the wording of the contract could not possibly have guaranteed a vaccine that was absolutely safe. He imagined a dialogue between a theoretical buyer and Cutter.

Buyer: I want some polio vaccine. What kind do you have?

Cutter: There is only one kind—the vaccine developed by Dr. Salk and licensed by the United States Public Health Service.

Buyer: Is this vaccine guaranteed to prevent polio?

Cutter: No. No medicine or vaccine is guaranteed to be 100 percent effective. Dr. Salk believes that it is substantially effective in preventing polio and that is why the United States Public Health Service has licensed it.

Buyer: Well, is it 100 percent safe? Is there any chance that I might get polio from the vaccine itself?

Cutter: Dr. Salk has assured us that this vaccine has a built-in factor of safety. In addition, we have tested it with the best available tests known to modern science at this time. The Public Health Service has licensed the vaccine and licensed this laboratory to produce it (and has specifically released each lot of vaccine) on the basis that, if its *Minimum Requirements* are followed, the vaccine will be safe. We have carefully followed those instructions; more than that we cannot say.

In his appeal to the district court, Sedgwick claimed that "there was no jury trial at all." The jury in its attachment to the verdict lamented that the judge had given it "no alternative" but to find Cutter liable. Sedgwick said, "The statement contained in the verdict . . . eloquently demonstrates that where the jury is made the prisoner of the court by rigid instructions it is deprived of its traditional fact-finding function and can only echo the trial court's own opinion."

Sedgwick used several examples to support his contention that the judge had bypassed the jury. By the late 1950s three lawsuits against Cutter Laboratories had gone to court. The judge in the third case, *Crane v. Cutter Laboratories*, gave instructions that were different from those given by Judge Ledwich in the Gottsdanker case. In the Crane case the judge said, "The product must be judged in the light of the scientific knowledge, skill, and experience available to the manufacturer *at the time it was produced and offered for sale.*" The jury, deadlocked six to six, was dismissed after three days of deliberation.

Also, by the late 1950s and early 1960s lawsuits had been filed against tobacco companies claiming that they should be held liable for harm caused by cigarettes. The first lawsuit was brought by the estate of Edwin Green, who died of lung cancer after smoking Lucky Strikes. His estate sued the makers of Lucky Strikes, the American Tobacco Company, for $1.5 million. At the time of the lawsuit it was clear that cigarette smoking caused lung cancer, but at the time that Edwin Green died, this association hadn't been proven. The judge asked the jury four questions:

(1) Did the decedent Green have primary cancer in his left lung?
(2) Was the cancer in his left lung the cause of his death?
(3) Was the smoking of Lucky Strike cigarettes a cause of cancer in his left lung?
(4) Could the defendant on or prior to February 1, 1956, have known that users of Lucky Strike cigarettes would contract cancer of the lung?

On August 2, 1960, the jury voted "yes" to the first three questions but "no" to the fourth question and found that the American Tobacco Company was not liable. In the early 1960s judges were not willing to subject tobacco companies to the tenet of liability without fault.

Sedgwick argued that liability without fault wouldn't make products safer if companies didn't know that their products were unsafe when they sold them: "Imposing liability on the manufacturer of new drugs and biologics will not reduce hazards; for one cannot guard against what lies beyond current scientific knowledge."

Sedgwick also argued that liability without fault would prevent pharmaceutical companies from developing new products: "These events [the Cutter Incident] were absolutely typical of the way medicine advances. Building on his predecessors and working in his laboratory, the researcher concludes that he has a useful product and tests it, realizing that every medicine, every new biologic, has risks and hazards. . . . Then the product must run the gamut of actual experience; experience leads to further research, research to alterations, and alterations to new experience."

Sedgwick wasn't alone. Statements by the editor of a prominent medical journal, the president of a major pharmaceutical company, and the director of a medical professional organization echoed his fears about the consequences of subjecting pharmaceutical companies to the tenet of liability without fault. "I am deeply disturbed about this decision," said Austin Smith, the editor of the *Journal of the American Medical Association*. "I have discussed it with . . . members of the [pharmaceutical] industry, with people who do research, and with a number of others who have no direct relationship to medicine. We all see in this decision a stepping stone to the creation of a fear so great that companies may no longer take a risk in developing new substances, researchers may be unwilling to try them in patients because of liability, and practicing doctors may even be afraid to give newer drugs for fear of the slight risk that may develop unexpectedly. I think this is far-reaching." E. N. Beesley, the president of Eli Lilly, said "The suggestion that the pharmaceutical industry should be subjected to the doctrine of liability without fault is a novel and shocking concept. In my opinion, its imposition would be a threat to the future of medicine and to the welfare of the people. [Acceptance of this principle] would delay, and even prevent, the introduction of many life-saving medicines. Who could afford to pioneer in pharmaceutical research? Who would dare to try anything new if it could mean undeserved ruin of their company?" The American College of Physicians, a nonprofit organization of ten thousand doctors, also expressed concern: "Few preventive or curative substances can, in the first instance, be both absolutely effective and absolutely harmless. Had the concept of absolute liability . . . been applied to biologics and drugs 200 years ago, Dr. Jenner and his colleagues would probably not have been able to make the giant contribution of the smallpox vaccine to mankind."

Finally, Sedgwick argued that if held to a standard of liability without fault, pharmaceutical companies would have trouble getting insurance, and the buyer would eventually pay a prohibitive price for their products: "Many of the advocates of unlimited compensation forget the ever increasing cost of such insurance can only be paid for by increasing the cost of the products involved, and hence must eventually be borne by the public."

Plaintiff's lawyers disagreed. In answering Sedgwick's brief, they argued that extending the law from foods to medical products was both logical and necessary. They argued that finding oyster shells in a can of oysters was different from finding live polio virus in a vial of polio vaccine: "Scientifically, medically, and in practical effect, live virus is the complete antithesis of a killed virus vaccine—the mixture of the two is like having bacteria in an antiseptic. How anyone can contend that this defect could possibly be a 'reasonable' imperfection under the circumstances is difficult . . . to understand."

They argued that defects were not acceptable as an industry standard when it meant that children would be paralyzed and killed: "Tacks in Coca-Cola, or [parasites] in sausage, or a lounging robe that catches fire are certainly products not of merchantable quality as a matter of law . . . but these defects may injure one, or maybe two, people, and the injuries, although severe, are not generally crippling. The 'defect' involved in these [Cutter] cases has been, in a tragic way, demonstrated to be both widespread and crippling."

They argued that development of new pharmaceutical products would not be hampered by the new standard of liability without fault: "Opponents of [liability without fault] argue that it tends to discourage people from performing socially advantageous activity that is accompanied by a high risk of loss. This 'stifling development' argument is, of course, presented at some stage of every lawsuit which in any way involves or relates to the medical and other scientific professions. That it has no merit at all in the product liability field is shown by the fact that the food industry, clearly subject to the highest degree of liability, has continually developed and marketed new food products."

They argued that Cutter was a business and should be treated like a business: "The remaining arguments and suggestions which are liberally sprinkled throughout the briefs on why the drug industry is deserving of special treatment from the courts would lead the unwary to believe that this Court was dealing with [a charitable] segment of American industry. This is, of course, not the case. The various drug-producing houses, Cutter included, are commercial enterprises, no more and no less. Cutter came into the polio program with no little eagerness as a commercial venture and, of course, its colleagues are still in the polio vaccine business to make a profit."

Finally, plaintiff's lawyers scoffed at the notion that pharmaceutical companies would have trouble getting insurance: "A word is in order on the argument that [liability without fault] 'will be too great and unpredictable in obtaining insurance coverage.' The point is absolutely absurd and the proof is not only that such coverage has been obtained universally in the food and drug business but that very substantial insurance coverage is present in the Cutter cases."

On July 12, 1960, Sedgwick's appeal to overturn the verdict in the Gottsdanker case was denied. On September 8, 1960, his appeal to the Supreme Court of the State of California was also denied.

Defendant's lawyers claimed that pharmaceutical companies would be unfairly crippled by the law of liability without fault. Plaintiff's lawyers claimed that making companies accountable for their products—even when they weren't negligent in producing those products—was necessary to protect the public's health. Events during the next fifty years would determine who was right.

Wallace Sedgwick argued that pharmaceutical companies should not be responsible for the process of trial and error required to make new products. He said that Cutter couldn't be "the guarantor of the scientifically unknowable, the warrantor of the future." But if medicine required knowledge gained at the expense of children's health—and sometimes at the expense of their lives—then who should warrant their future? Was it fair to require that Anne Gottsdanker buy insurance to protect her from polio caused by a polio vaccine? Or was it more reasonable to require the company that made the vaccine, or the government that recommended it, to provide that insurance for her? By making pharmaceutical companies financially responsible for their products, even when they weren't negligent in producing them, the courts decided that it was the vaccine makers that should insure Anne against harm.

The framers of this revolution in product liability law imagined the following scenario: Companies would continue to make new products. Products would be tested in hundreds of people and, if safe and effective, would be licensed by federal regulators. Because rare problems might not be found until after licensure (only one of every fifteen hundred people given Cutter's vaccine was paralyzed), companies would buy more insurance and the cost of that insurance would be passed on to the consumer. Everyone who bought the product, and therefore everyone who benefited from its use, would pay a "liability tax" on all medical products.

In 1955, only months after Anne Gottsdanker was paralyzed by Cutter's vaccine, an article entitled "The Cutter Vaccine Incident" appeared in the *Yale Law Journal*. The article predicted the coming revolution: "[The courts should] establish clearly that manufacturers of products for human consumption are liable for personal injuries caused by their products, not because they are at 'fault' for the injuries, nor because they would have prevented them, but because they can best distribute this unavoidable cost to all persons who benefit from the enterprise." The authors of the article were saying that it didn't matter who was wrong, why they were wrong, or whether the wrong was predictable. The only thing that mattered was who was in the best position to pay when products caused harm. The revolution triggered by the Gottsdanker decision determined exactly who would pay. The price of liability without fault would not be borne by the government, by pharmaceutical companies, or by insurance companies—it would be borne by every person who bought a given product. The article predicted that this liability tax would make for better, safer products: "[Liability without fault will] provide the producer with added incentive to prevent avoidable defects in the future."

Wallace Sedgwick argued that if Cutter Laboratories were subjected to a standard of liability without fault, it would not survive.

What happened to Cutter Laboratories in the years following the trag-edy? Sixty lawsuits were filed against Cutter, but only a few went to court. Although claims totaled $12 million, plaintiffs settled for $3 million; $2 million was paid by Cutter's existing insurance, and the rest was paid by Cutter out of pocket. Despite its setback, Cutter had no trouble borrowing money, acquiring companies, or expanding fa-cilities. Within months of the tragedy Wells Fargo Bank extended Cut-ter's line of credit to $1 million, and Mutual of New York agreed to a $3 million loan. Between 1955 and 1961 Cutter launched "Operation Comeback."

In 1955 Cutter purchased Ashe-Lockhart, Inc. and Haver-Glover Laboratories. Both were located in Kansas City, and both manufac-tured veterinary products. The purchase of these two firms allowed Cutter to add three hundred new products to its line. Cutter also purchased Plastron Specialties, a plastics company, for the manufac-ture of bottles and tubing used in its intravenous solutions business. Annual sales for Cutter Laboratories in 1955 were $11,482,000. In 1956 Cutter hired Marcus Van Campen from the Merrell Company of Cincinnati, Ohio, to head its expanded research operations. It also bought another plastics firm, Pacific Plastics Company of San Fran-cisco, as well as an animal feed firm, the Corn King Company of Cedar Rapids, Iowa. Annual sales increased to $13,731,000. In 1957 Cutter built a new pharmacology and organic research building. "Operation Comeback is really succeeding," said Robert Cutter. Annual sales in-creased to $16,185,000. In 1958 Cutter bought Hollister-Stier, manu-facturers of allergy products with factories in Spokane, Los Angeles, Philadelphia, and Atlanta. Cutter's product line grew, and annual sales increased to $18,745,000. In 1959 Cutter bought Olympic Plastics Company of Los Angeles. "Another record year for Cutter Laborato-ries!" Robert Cutter declared. Cutter also established Cutter Labora-tories Pacific, Inc., in Japan and appointed Walter Ward head of Japa-nese research operations. Annual sales increased to $21,315,000. In 1960 the second case against Cutter Laboratories, on behalf of four children paralyzed by the vaccine, concluded with a jury award of $120,000. The third case, *Crane v. Cutter Laboratories*, was settled for $189,000. Annual sales increased to $23 million.

Cutter went to trial four times. Juries never found that Cutter was negligent, and Cutter eventually settled all other cases pending against it. The largest settlement against Cutter Laboratories, $600,000, was in the case of Brian May. May, who was five years old when he was injected with Cutter's vaccine, spent sixteen months in an iron lung and was a quadriplegic for the rest of his life. May's lawyer, Melvin Belli, remembered, "It was up to that time, the highest personal injury award in history. Today [1976], that verdict would easily have gone $6 million or more." In his thirties, Brian May hosted a radio program in Los Angeles called "Malibu Folk" that featured interviews with musicians such as Peter Yarrow and Gordon Lightfoot. After his death in 1995, May was remembered as "one of acoustic music's true angels."

In 1961 Robert Cutter summarized events following the polio vaccine tragedy in a letter to stockholders:

> We have licked a nightmare! We have come through our polio vaccine difficulties with integrity and with financial soundness.
>
> Seven years ago, come April 27, we have faced the possibility that our polio vaccine might have caused polio.
>
> From that day on, those of us who have responsibility for the affairs of the Laboratories never awakened in the morning without the feeling that this possibility must be a "bad dream," and with these awakening thoughts was the terrific weight of undetermined financial liability, to say nothing of our heartfelt concern for the children and the families involved.
>
> And so, each day and each week, we worked to make our company strong enough to be able to pay what might possibly be assessed against us in the final reckoning.
>
> The key to our whole problem was whether we could borrow sufficient money to carry us through when the $2,000,000 insurance money was exhausted. Furthermore, our long-term loan agreement had provisions which restricted our borrowing such a large sum.
>
> So we put the problem to the lenders. Our bankers told us that, if settlements could be held to fair and reasonable amounts, they would support us.
>
> Had we not done so much to improve our financial strength and future prospects between 1955 and 1961, it is clear that these financial institutions could not have supported us—and without this support we were dead ducks.
>
> This means that for all practical purposes, our polio difficulties are behind us and now we can go on to a future which we expect to make bright.
>
> For one who has not gone through it, it is inconceivable to realize the degree to which this polio situation has clouded every decision we have made.
>
> Now, for the first time in seven years, we can make decisions on their own merits.

In 1961 Cutter's annual sales increased to $24,808,000. "Never has the future looked brighter," Robert Cutter declared. One of the products developed by Cutter's new director of research, Marcus Van Campen, was an analgesic (pain medicine). Cutter didn't have the money to directly promote this drug to the public, so it licensed the patent to Bristol-Myers, who named it Excedrin. By the early 1960s Cutter was receiving substantial royalty checks from the sales of Excedrin.

In 1962, after recorded annual sales of $29,934,000, Robert Cutter said, "What a 'grand and glorious feeling!' We made a record high in sales, earnings, and in earnings per share." The company's assets, $18,300,000, were 80 percent greater than when the polio vaccine disaster occurred. Melvin Belli watched Cutter thrive after the tragedy. "Did it break Cutter? Hell, no!" he said. By 1963 market analysts were recommending the purchase of Cutter stock "for substantial long-term capital gains." In the early 1960s Cutter's catalogue included more than seven hundred products. Sedgwick's dire predictions of Cutter's fate were wrong.

Wallace Sedgwick was also wrong when he predicted that liability without fault would deny medical research the luxury of trial and error. Several difficult vaccines—like those for measles, mumps, and German measles—were quickly developed. The utopian world envisioned by the plaintiff lawyers in the Cutter cases and by those who had contributed to the article in the *Yale Law Journal* was realized. "The decision didn't hurt business or consumers," said Belli. "Since then, the pharmaceutical industry has gone ahead with their pioneering medicine—to the health of the public and, I must add quietly, the swelling of their own purses."

During the next fifty years, however, two critical flaws in the system were exposed.

By no longer requiring personal injury lawyers to prove negligence, companies were more easily held liable for products that were harmful. They were also more easily held liable for products that were safe.

In 1956 the Merrell Company (later Merrell Dow) introduced Bendectin, a drug for morning sickness (the severe nausea and vomiting of early pregnancy). The drug consisted of doxylamine (an antihistamine), pyridoxine (vitamin B_6), and dicyclomine hydrochloride (an antispasmodic to calm the stomach). From the 1950s through the 1970s Bendectin, used in up to 40 percent of all pregnancies in the United States, was the only medicine available to relieve morning sickness. Morning sickness wasn't a trivial problem. During early pregnancy, women, unable to replenish fluids lost because of frequent and persistent vomiting, would suffer severe and occasionally fatal dehydration. In 1855 Charlotte Brontë, the author of *Jane Eyre,* died from morning sickness.

In 1979 the *National Enquirer,* under the headline "New Thalidomide Scandal—Experts Reveal," stated, "In a monstrous scandal that could be far larger than the thalidomide horror, untold thousands of babies are being born with hideous defects after their mothers took an anti-nausea drug (Bendectin) during early pregnancy." The article stated that the medical term for drugs that caused birth defects was "teratogen," literally "the formation or bringing forth of monsters." Information for the *Enquirer*'s story was provided by Melvin Belli. In response to the story, as Belli hoped, many women stepped forward claiming that their babies had been deformed by Bendectin.

Before Bendectin was available, about 2 percent of all children born in the United States had birth defects. If 40 percent of pregnant women used Bendectin then by chance alone one would predict that about twenty thousand children with birth defects would be born every year to women who had taken Bendectin. This didn't mean that Bendectin caused birth defects. The only way to determine whether Bendectin was the culprit was to compare the incidence of birth defects in children whose mothers had taken Bendectin with that in mothers who hadn't. Twenty-seven separate studies examined the incidence of birth defects in pregnancies where Bendectin had or hadn't been used. All reached the same conclusion: Bendectin didn't cause birth defects.

On January 24, 1980, in a courtroom in Orlando, Florida, lawyers tried the first case against Merrell Dow on behalf of David Mekdeci, a child who was born with a malformed arm and a deformity of his chest. In the absence of scientific studies showing that Bendectin caused harm, the jury found that Merrell Dow was not responsible for David's deformities. But the Mekdeci case didn't discourage lawyers from suing Merrell Dow. In February 1982 lawyers on behalf of Mary Oxendine, a child born with a shortened forearm and three fingers fused together on her right hand, sued Merrell Dow for $20 million. After a three-week trial—which included scientific evidence that Bendectin didn't cause birth defects—the jury awarded Mary $750,000.

Pregnant women were caught in the middle of the controversy. Doctors were saying that Bendectin was safe, but the courts, by occasionally finding Merrell Dow guilty, were saying that Bendectin was unsafe. At least seven women, terrified that they had harmed their unborn children by taking Bendectin, aborted their babies. Many women desperately sought alternatives. Dr. Gary Ritchwald, in an article in the popular magazine *Mother Jones,* advised pregnant women to take "natural alternatives" to Bendectin that included "vitamin B_6 (50–100 mg), vitamin B_1 (100 mg), wild yam root, raspberry leaf, peppermint, chamomile, lemon balm, catnip, comfrey tea, honey, and herbal teas." Ironically, the quantity of vitamin B_6 in Dr. Ritchwald's mixture was ten times more than that in Bendectin, and unlike Bendectin, none of his remedies had been studied in pregnant women and found to be safe.

Heartened by the Oxendine verdict, law firms launched publicity campaigns, and the number of Bendectin lawsuits increased. In 1987 a jury awarded $2 million to a boy with clubfeet. By July 1987 seventeen juries had considered Bendectin cases; Merrell Dow won twelve times, and plaintiffs won five times. Merrell Dow spent $120 million defending these lawsuits. The combination of the *National Enquirer* article and sympathetic stories in *Mother Jones* and the *New York Times* caused sales of Bendectin to drop to one-fifth of what they had been. On June 9, 1983, Merrell Dow stopped making Bendectin. Later, because of overwhelming scientific evidence showing that Bendectin never caused birth defects, all five cases in favor of the plaintiffs were overturned on appeal. But it was too late; by that time, Bendectin was already off the market. A spokesman for Merrell Dow said, "We wouldn't bring Bendectin back if we won every lawsuit." The Bendectin litigation has been called the "Taj Mahal of horror stories about the tort system."

In addition to the problem that companies could now be held liable for safe products, a second flaw in the system was that there were no limits on the amounts of money that could be awarded to plaintiffs. Companies couldn't learn to make safer products if they were forced to go out of business. For example, in 1992 David Kessler, director of the Food and Drug Administration, decided that there was insufficient evidence that silicone-filled breast implants were safe. At the time, breast implants had been on the market for thirty years and had been used by 2 million Americans. Most were used for augmentation, but about 20 percent were used as prostheses following breast removal (mastectomy) for cancer. Although silicone-filled breast implants had not been shown to be unsafe, Kessler asked manufacturers to withdraw them from the market.

Kessler's ban precipitated an onslaught of litigation. Personal injury lawyers advertised for clients, and the number of lawsuits directed against the principal manufacturer, Dow Corning, increased from two hundred in 1991 to ten thousand in 1992. Women with silicone-filled breast implants claimed a variety of symptoms including fever, headache, fatigue, rash, joint pains, muscle aches, dry eyes and mouth, and disturbed sleep—symptoms that taken together constituted what were called connective-tissue diseases.

Lawyers consolidated thousands of cases and in 1994 settled the largest class-action lawsuit in history—$4.25 billion. That same year, Sherine Gabriel reported the results of the first study. Gabriel examined the medical records of 750 women who had had breast implants and compared them with 1,500 women who hadn't. She made sure that the two groups were comparable in age, race, income, marital status, smoking history, and medical background. Because these two groups were comparable in all medical aspects—with the exception of receiving or not receiving breast implants—the effect of the implants could be determined. Gabriel found "no association between breast implants and connective-tissue diseases." One year later Gabriel's findings were duplicated by Jorge Sanchez-Guerrero, who studied 90,000 nurses, 1,200 of whom had received breast implants. Again, women who had received breast implants were not at greater risk of connective-tissue diseases than those who hadn't. During the next two years, six more studies found the same thing: breast implants didn't cause connective-tissue diseases.

Plaintiff's lawyers in the case of *Gottsdanker v. Cutter Laboratories* had claimed that liability without fault was necessary to protect the public's health. But because silicone-filled breast implants didn't cause connective-tissue diseases, the $4.25 billion given by Dow Corning to lawyers and plaintiffs didn't reduce the incidence of connective-tissue diseases and didn't make breast implants safer. In 1999 the Institute of Medicine, in a 530-page document reviewing all published studies, concluded that breast implants didn't cause chronic diseases. Dow Corning had already filed for bankruptcy.

In the cases of Bendectin and breast implants the courts weren't performing their most important function—to act as a deterrent to companies that produced unsafe products. After their court cases the companies that made Bendectin and breast implants didn't become more attentive to making safer products because their products weren't unsafe; they were just found to be unsafe in court.

Consumers also suffered. Dr. Charles Flowers, vice president of the American College of Obstetricians and Gynecologists, lamented the decision by Merrell Dow to stop making Bendectin. "The decision of Merrell Dow creates a significant therapeutic gap," said Flowers. "Nausea and vomiting in pregnancy cannot always be treated by symptomatic means, and in past years severe cases have led to serious maternal nutritional deficiencies and nerve damage. We understand the Merrell Dow decision in view of the present legal climate. This decision is made on the basis of law instead of science." Flowers's words rang true. By the end of the 1980s, because no medicine had replaced (or dared to replace) Bendectin, the incidence of hospitalization for dehydration during pregnancy doubled; the incidence of birth defects was unchanged. Bendectin has never been replaced.

But the Bendectin decision went well beyond Bendectin. One year after Bendectin was taken off the market, the president of a major pharmaceutical company asked, "Who in his right mind would work on a product today that would be used by a pregnant woman?" This question was an ominous predictor of future events. Because of liability fears, pharmaceutical companies continue to avoid the two biggest problems of pregnancy: miscarriage and morning sickness.

Judges, juries, doctors, lawyers, and plaintiffs each play a part in finding pharmaceutical companies liable when scientific studies find that their products are not harmful. Judges, with little training in science or the scientific method, are often poor arbiters of scientific truths. On July 1, 1981, Katie Wells was born with birth defects that included deformities of her hand, arm, shoulder, lip, nose, and optic nerve (the nerve that connects the eye to the brain). For several weeks after conception—not realizing that she was already pregnant—Katie's mother used the spermicidal jelly OrthoGynol, a product made by Ortho Pharmaceuticals. The active ingredient in OrthoGynol was Nonoxynol-9. In 1986 Katie Wells's parents sued Ortho Pharmaceuticals claiming that Nonoxynol-9 had caused their daughter's birth defects. In 1982, four years before the lawsuit, a paper in the *Journal of the American Medical Association* had reported the outcomes of 50,300 pregnancies. Comparing pregnancies where Nonoxynol-9 had been used after conception with those where it hadn't researchers found that Nonoxynol-9 didn't cause arm, shoulder, hand, lip, or optic nerve defects; indeed, Nonoxynol-9 didn't cause any major or minor birth defects. Two other studies by the Food and Drug Administration also found no evidence that Nonoxynol-9 caused birth defects. But the judge at the Wells trial, Marvin Shoob, unimpressed by the scientific data, decided that the deformities of Katie's arm, shoulder, and hand had been caused by Nonoxynol-9 and that her lip, nose, and optic nerve defects hadn't. On what evidence he based this decision is unknown. There were no studies at the time and remain no studies today that support the ruling. Shoob awarded Katie Wells $5.1 million, a judgment upheld by a federal court of appeals.

An editorial in the *New York Times* lamented judge Shoob's decision: "Science's finest achievement is finding methods to raise objective evidence above the merely anecdotal. Judge Shoob was not moved by the preponderance of scientific evidence—and neither was the appeals court. That Judge Shoob and the appellate judges ignored the best scientific evidence is an intellectual embarrassment." An editorial in the *New England Journal of Medicine* also worried about the rejection of science in the courtroom: "The *Wells v. Ortho* decisions are of great concern to the medical community because they indicate that the courts will not be bound by reasonable scientific standards of proof."

Jurors are also not usually well suited to decide complicated issues of medicine, science, and technology. In 1986 Judith Haimes had a CT scan of her head at Temple University Hospital in Philadelphia. (A CT [computerized tomography] scan is a detailed X-ray that visualizes cross-sections of the brain.) Haimes, a psychic who made her living predicting the future and contacting the dead, found that soon after the CT scan, her psychic powers were gone. She sued her doctor for damages. For the jury to find the doctor guilty it would need to be convinced of three things: first, that people have psychic powers to lose; second, that they can lose these powers in a CT scanner; and third, that a doctor should know better than to order a CT scan on a psychic. On March 27, 1986, after deliberating for forty-five minutes, an eight-person jury found the doctor negligent and awarded Judith Haimes $986,000.

Jurors such as those selected for the Haimes jury are randomly selected from voter registration pools. They are often asked to determine whether vaccines, airplanes, lawn mowers, drugs, trampolines, and diving boards are made and tested correctly. Because jurors—and not those who regulate and license products—are the final arbiters in the courtroom, they are presumed to know more than pharmacologists and microbiologists at the Food and Drug Administration; more than epidemiologists and statisticians at the Centers for Disease Control and Prevention; more than toxicologists at the Environmental Protection Agency; and more than mechanical engineers at the Federal Aviation Administration. Unfortunately, jurors often have little experience with or understanding of science, so they tend to believe whoever seems to be the most believable. If a plaintiff's expert witness is well dressed, well spoken, and interacts comfortably with the jury (but has little credible data to support his contention) and the defense witness is shy, bookish, soft-spoken, cautious, and hesitant (but has a wealth of data to support his contention), the jury is likely to be more impressed with the plaintiff's case. In the Bendectin lawsuits 30 percent of juries found in favor of the plaintiffs even though not one expert showed that Bendectin caused birth defects.

Jurors also have an enormous amount of sympathy for someone who is suffering, and sympathy can cloud their ability to evaluate science dispassionately. Mary Oxendine was eleven years old when she sat in the courtroom with a shortened arm and weblike hand and looked across the table at several well-dressed senior executives from the Merrell Dow Company. It is not hard to understand how—even in the presence of solid science disputing her claim—the jury could find on Mary's behalf. In one early Bendectin case, the jury, convinced by the data presented, ruled that Merrell Dow was not liable—but it still wanted the company to pay the plaintiff $20,000 to cover medical expenses.

Doctors have also been willing to say things in court that are not supported by scientific studies. The star witness for the plaintiffs in the case against Merrell Dow and Bendectin was William McBride, an Australian obstetrician. McBride was an impressive presence in the courtroom. In the early 1960s he was the first physician to notice a sudden increase in an extremely rare birth defect following the use of a popular sleeping pill. The sleeping pill was made by the West German pharmaceutical company Chemie Grünenthal. In 1954 chemists at Grünenthal made a compound called thalidomide. To their disappointment they found that thalidomide wasn't an antibiotic and in animal tests had no anti-tumor effect. The drug was a bust. But in a small clinical trial in humans thalidomide put patients into a deep, all-night, "natural" sleep. On October 1, 1957, Grünenthal distributed thalidomide as a sleeping pill and advertised it as completely safe, even for pregnant women and nursing mothers. By 1960 hundreds of babies were born with their hands and feet directly attached to their bodies— a disorder called phocomelia—following the mother's use of thalidomide. McBride was the first to describe this association in a medical journal. As many as twenty-four thousand embryos were damaged by thalidomide, and nearly half died before birth. Today, five thousand people live with birth defects caused by thalidomide.

McBride, with his thalidomide fame behind him, felt that Bendectin also caused birth defects. His claim was based on a paper that he published in the *Australian Journal of Biological Science* describing eight pregnant rabbits inoculated with the drug scopolamine; eight untreated rabbits served as controls. McBride found that rabbits fed scopolamine delivered babies with birth defects and that rabbits not fed scopolamine delivered normal babies. Although Bendectin didn't contain scopolamine, McBride argued that the antihistamine in Bendectin (doxylamine) was similar. At the time that McBride submitted his paper, the two co-authors, Phil Vardy and Jill French, requested that their names be removed because they believed that McBride had knowingly falsified data. The Medical Tribunal in Australia investigated their charges and found them to be true and, as a consequence, McBride resigned his position. McBride was later stripped of his medical license and never testified in subsequent trials of Bendectin. Another expert in the Bendectin lawsuits, Dr. Alan Done, testified that he was a professor of toxicology at Wayne State University when no such position existed. Done, who had a lucrative consulting business as an expert witness, was later asked by the dean of his school to resign because he was neglecting his academic duties.

The Bendectin trials weren't the first time that doctors had been willing to lie in court. In the early 1900s workers' compensation laws were established in Germany and later in the United States. These laws set aside money to compensate workers for accidents and established a large and tempting pool of money for personal injury lawyers. Workers claimed that their cancers had been caused by traumatic injuries. They claimed that stomach cancer had been caused by a fight with a police officer (1923); that rib cancer had been caused by a fall from an elevator shaft (1927); that breast cancer had been caused by a blow from a can of orange juice (1949); that bone cancer had been caused by heavy lifting (1958); that testicular cancer had been caused by a seat belt during a sudden stop (1963); and that lung cancer had been caused by a chest bruise (1964). Although no data existed to support these claims, doctors testified in court that trauma caused cancer. Many studies have since shown that trauma doesn't cause cancer. The British courts eliminate the problem of "experts" willing to say anything for the right price by hiring independent experts to determine the legitimacy of plaintiff's claims.

In some ways, lawyers and scientists are alike. Both form a hypothesis—for example, "Bendectin causes birth defects"—and both establish burdens of proof to support or reject the hypothesis. For scientists proof comes with scientific studies that compare the outcomes of pregnancies in thousands of women who used Bendectin with thousands who did not. Differences are then subjected to statistical analysis. If the incidence of birth defects is greater in the group that took Bendectin and the differences are statistically significant, then the investigator can say that Bendectin caused birth defects. If the differences between the two groups are not statistically significant, then the investigator can say that the data do not support the hypothesis. If many investigators evaluating different populations of women find the same result, then a "truth" emerges. Sometimes it takes months, years, or even decades before a certain truth emerges. Sometimes it never emerges.

The difference between lawyers and scientists is at the level of proof. The goal of lawyers is to convince a jury that a claim is correct, and they assemble medical experts who will support their claim. "Truth," determined by a vote of the jury, is declared in a few weeks. If the jury votes that Bendectin caused birth defects, then Bendectin caused birth defects. Russ Herman, former president of the Association of Trial Lawyers of America, said, "The courts are an institution established for the resolution of disputes, not arbiters of scientific truth. History shows that many 'facts' lack staying power." However, the facts that Bendectin didn't cause birth defects, that breast implants didn't cause connective-tissue diseases, and that trauma didn't cause cancer have proven to be maddeningly stubborn.

Finally, some plaintiffs sue because they assume that no one will be hurt—that is, doctors, hospitals, and pharmaceutical companies have vast resources, and those resources can be relinquished without consequence. But we all pay for the cost of lawsuits. "We sue the stranger . . . as if we are disconnected from the implications of the suit," says Peter Huber, a lawyer who writes extensively about abuses of the tort system. "In the short run, and for a small minority of successful litigation, conflict is a profitable business. But in the longer run, as society adjusts to a legal regime that promotes division, everyone loses but the lawyers. We are all in the soup together. Only the lawyers are here to dine."

9

Death for the Lambs

Liberty for the wolves is death for the lambs.
—Isaiah Berlin

THE CUTTER INCIDENT HAS MANY LEGACIES. FOR one thing, the incident led to the effective federal regulation of vaccines. Because Cutter Laboratories made a vaccine that caused paralysis, the federal government launched an immediate investigation into the manufacture and testing procedures of all companies; it found that regulations and guidelines were inadequate. Better procedures for filtration, storage, and safety testing were developed, and within months safe polio vaccine was made. Within a few years, the number of children paralyzed or killed by natural polio decreased by a factor of ten. On July 15, 1955, only three months after the incident, the Laboratory of Biologics Control became the Division of Biologic Standards, a separate division within the National Institutes of Health. By 1956 the number of professionals regulating vaccines increased from 10 to 150, and regulators were actively involved in studying the vaccines that they supervised. A series of consecutive lots of vaccine that are equal in potency, safety, and efficacy continues to be required of all vaccine makers, and the term "consistency lots," born of the Cutter Incident, is still used.

In 1972 vaccine regulation moved from the National Institutes of Health to the Food and Drug Administration (FDA). The FDA now employs more than 250 people to monitor the design and manufacture of vaccines. Vaccines undergo thousands of tests to make sure that they contain exactly what they are said to contain; they are tested in tens of thousands of people before they are licensed to make sure that they are safe and that they work; and they are watched very carefully after licensure—when they are given to millions of people—to make sure that they don't cause any rare side effects. Vaccines are arguably held to a higher standard of safety than any other product given to children, including antibiotics and cough and cold preparations. As a consequence, during the past fifty years, vaccines have had a record of safety matched by no other medical product. Today the percentage of children in the United States immunized with vaccines is the highest in history, and as a consequence, the incidence of vaccine-preventable diseases is the lowest.

The Cutter Incident was also the "first coordinated national response to a public health emergency" in the history of the United States, caused a massive infusion of money into Alexander Langmuir's Epidemic Intelligence Service, and was a turning point in the history of the Centers for Disease Control and Prevention (CDC). Since the inception of the Epidemic Intelligence Service, its officers, dramatized in movies such as *And the Band Played On* and *Outbreak,* have monitored diseases such as anthrax, Severe Acute Respiratory Syndrome (SARS), smallpox, and influenza and have determined how specific diseases—most notably Acquired Immune Deficiency Syndrome (AIDS)—spread.

But perhaps Cutter's most enduring legacy is the birth of liability without fault for pharmaceutical companies. Because of the ruling in *Gottsdanker v. Cutter Laboratories,* vaccines were among the first medical products almost eliminated by lawsuits. Initially unaffected by the Gottsdanker verdict, difficult vaccines, such as those for measles and German measles (rubella), were tested and sold. In the mid-1970s, however, one vaccine changed everything.

In 1974 a British researcher co-authored a paper claiming that the pertussis (whooping cough) vaccine caused permanent brain damage. Pertussis was a common disease of young children. The bacteria caused thick, sticky mucus to accumulate on the back of the throat and block the windpipe. Children with whooping cough often had spasms of coughing so severe that they turned blue; when they tried to breathe in against a narrowed windpipe, they made a high-pitched, distinctive whooping sound. In the first half of the twentieth century, between five thousand and ten thousand infants and young children in the United States died every year from whooping cough; typically they died from suffocation.

In his article the British researcher reported the stories of thirty-six children: one or two days after receiving the pertussis vaccine, all had seizures, limpness, vomiting, screaming, or extreme irritability. Among these children, twenty-two eventually developed mental retardation or a seizure disorder (epilepsy). Although millions of children received the pertussis vaccine every year without consequence, the report claimed that the vaccine caused permanent brain damage. At the time the article was published, 80 percent of children in the United Kingdom received pertussis vaccine; also mental retardation and epilepsy had occurred in children even before the vaccine was available. So the only way to determine whether the British researcher was right was to examine the incidence of mental retardation and epilepsy in children who had received the vaccine and compare it with those who hadn't. Unfortunately the media in England—failing to appreciate the difference between proposing a theory about a vaccine and proving that a vaccine was harmful—seized upon the publication as fact. Urgent reports in the media warned of permanent brain damage owing to the vaccine, and most parents stopped giving it to their children. Immunization rates dropped from 80 to 30 percent, and within two years more than one hundred thousand children in England were hospitalized and forty killed by pertussis.

Media coverage of the pertussis story traveled to Japan. In 1975 the Japanese minister of health, responding to a public outcry, declared that Japanese children would no longer receive the pertussis vaccine. The incidence of hospitalization and death from pertussis increased tenfold. Between 1976 and 1979, 113 children in Japan died from pertussis; in the three years before the vaccine was discontinued, only ten had died from the disease.

Stories that pertussis vaccine harmed children soon appeared in the United States, and personal injury lawyers attacked vaccine makers, claiming that the pertussis vaccine caused epilepsy, mental retardation, learning disorders, unexplained coma, Reye's syndrome (a sudden onset of coma, later found to be associated with aspirin), and sudden infant death syndrome (sudden unexplained death in the first year of life, later found to be associated with sleep position). By 1987 eight hundred lawsuits totaling more than $21 million had been filed, and new claims were filed every week. To meet the demand for increased liability insurance and to pay for legal fees and settlements, the cost of the pertussis vaccine increased from $0.17 to $11.00 per dose.

By the late 1980s and early 1990s many scientists had examined the question raised by the British researcher; they evaluated hundreds of thousands of children who did or did not receive pertussis vaccine in several different countries. The results were clear, consistent, and reproducible: the incidence of epilepsy and mental retardation in children who had received pertussis vaccine was the same as in those who hadn't. The British researcher's hypothesis was wrong, but the damage was done. The number of companies making pertussis vaccine for children in the United States decreased from four (Wyeth, Connaught, Sclavo, and Lederle) to one (Lederle).

In the mid-1980s Lederle was punished for its persistence. In 1979 three-month-old Kevin Toner received a pertussis vaccine made by Lederle. Soon after receipt of the vaccine, because of inflammation of one segment of his spinal cord, Kevin was completely and permanently paralyzed below the waist. Kevin's parents sued Lederle, claiming that the pertussis vaccine had paralyzed their son. Lederle had several facts on its side: the incidence of children with spinal cord swelling didn't increase after the pertussis vaccine was first introduced in the United States in the early 1940s; children immunized with pertussis vaccine didn't have a higher incidence of spinal cord swelling than unimmunized children; and natural infection with pertussis bacteria didn't damage the spinal cord. But in the courtroom, science didn't matter. The jury ruled against Lederle and awarded Kevin Toner $1.13 million. At the time of the award, gross sales from the pertussis vaccine in the United States were about $2 million, and gross sales from all vaccines were about $7 million.

The case of *Toner v. Lederle Laboratories* showed exactly what can happen when unanticipated events occur. The framers of the revolution in liability law reasoned that pharmaceutical companies should pay for harm caused by their products because by increasing the price of the product, they were in the best position to defray the cost of increased insurance. But the framers didn't predict how massive those awards would become, and they didn't predict that awards would be made when products weren't harmful. The award in the Toner case was the equivalent of one-half of the pertussis vaccine market in the mid-1980s. Pharmaceutical companies looked at this situation and decided to leave the vaccine business. The revolution in liability law—designed to coerce companies to make safer products by threatening financial punishment—was causing companies to abandon safe products vital to the nation's health.

Threatened by a return to the pre-vaccine era—when hundreds of thousands of children were routinely hospitalized, permanently harmed, or killed by vaccine-preventable diseases—the government stepped forward. In 1986 Congress passed the National Childhood Vaccine Injury Act. The heart of the act was the National Vaccine Injury Compensation Program, designed to protect companies from lawsuits not supported by scientific evidence; the program was funded by a federal excise tax on every dose of vaccine. In many ways, the vaccine compensation program was a model system to prevent abuses by personal injury lawyers. Scientists, epidemiologists, virologists, microbiologists, clinicians, and statisticians reviewed scientific studies and recommended to the courts which problems were caused by vaccines and which coincidentally followed vaccines. If a child suffered a reaction caused by a vaccine, the program was designed to compensate the family for medical expenses and damages quickly, generously, and fairly.

Unfortunately, despite protections afforded by the National Vaccine Injury Compensation Program, pharmaceutical companies are gradually abandoning vaccines. In 1957, when Cutter Laboratories made a vaccine that wasn't safe, twenty-six companies were making five vaccines. In 1980, when the first lawsuits against the makers of pertussis vaccine were filed, seventeen companies were making eight vaccines. In 2004 four big companies (GlaxoSmithKline, Sanofi-Aventis, Merck, and Wyeth) were making twelve vaccines. Although some of this decrease can be accounted for by merger, most is the result of dropouts. For example, Eli Lilly and Parke-Davis—the two large companies that made Jonas Salk's polio vaccine for the 1954 field trial—eventually abandoned vaccines. Of the twelve vaccines routinely given to young children, seven are made by a single manufacturer; only one vaccine is made by more than two companies. Because fewer companies make vaccines, limited supplies and scant reserves are available to meet a crisis. Events surrounding the influenza vaccine between 2003 and 2005 are particularly instructive.

The news media rarely report the yearly epidemic of influenza in the United States, but in 2003 the epidemic started early, and television reports of children dying from the disease were common. People were desperate to get an influenza vaccine. Unfortunately only one big pharmaceutical company, Aventis, made it. In 2003 Aventis made 48 million doses, and Chiron, a small British vaccine manufacturer, made 35 million doses. When the epidemic hit, the number of people who demanded vaccine greatly exceeded the supply. Because reserves were small, a vaccine shortage resulted. Many people who wanted and needed the influenza vaccine early in the epidemic couldn't get it. Between October 2003 and April 2004, 36,000 people died from influenza; 152 were children.

Problems with the influenza vaccine continued one year later. In 2004 Aventis made 55 million doses, and Chiron, in an effort to avoid the shortfall in 2003, made 48 million doses. But Chiron had a manufacturing problem, and all 48 million doses were withdrawn before the start of the influenza season. As a consequence, the United States entered the 2004 season knowing that about 30 million people who had been immunized the previous year would not be receiving influenza vaccine. The CDC, the FDA, and pharmaceutical companies were all blamed for inefficiency, and during the presidential debates on October 13, 2004, both candidates accused each other of failing to provide the nation with needed vaccine.

The shortage of influenza vaccine is just one example in what has been a steady, unrelenting procession of vaccine shortages. Between 1998 and 2004 severe shortages occurred for the diphtheria, tetanus, pertussis, measles, mumps, rubella (German measles), pneumococcal, influenza, and varicella (chickenpox) vaccines; there have been shortages in nine of the twelve vaccines routinely recommended for all children. Every one of these shortages resulted in a delay in the receipt of vaccines, and some children never caught up when vaccine became available.

The pneumococcal vaccine shortage was particularly damaging.

First licensed in the United States in 2000, the pneumococcal vaccine protects children against disease caused by pneumococcal bacteria. Before the vaccine was available in the United States, every year pneumococcus caused tens of thousands of cases of severe pneumonia, meningitis, and bloodstream infections in young children. Thousands of children died or were left with permanent brain damage because of pneumococcus. Only one company (Wyeth) makes the pneumococcal vaccine for children. By August 2004 the shortage of pneumococcal vaccine was so severe that the CDC recommended rationing it. Instead of the recommended four doses in the first and second years of life, the CDC recommended that children receive only two doses. Although studies showed that a four-dose schedule clearly prevented pneumococcal infections, a two-dose schedule had never been tested to see if it worked. In mid-2004 a sixteen-month-old boy was hospitalized in Philadelphia with severe pneumonia caused by pneumococcus. His parents had been told by their pediatrician that he couldn't get all four doses of the pneumococcal vaccine because of the shortage. Despite adequate antibiotic therapy and heroic supportive measures, the boy's pneumonia worsened, and he died from the disease. The pneumococcus isolated from the child's blood was a type that could have been prevented by the vaccine. If the vaccine were made by several companies, children wouldn't have to rely on the production efficiency of one company to save their lives.

The National Vaccine Injury Compensation Program was designed to keep pharmaceutical companies in the vaccine business by protecting them from abuses by personal injury lawyers, but the program has several weaknesses that hurt vaccine makers and, as a consequence, the public. The biggest weakness in the program is that plaintiffs can easily opt out of it. The program pays only for problems that are caused by vaccines; it does not pay for problems that are not caused by vaccines. When the program rejects claims not supported by scientific and medical studies, lawyers often choose to take their chances in front of a jury. Probably the best example is the case against thimerosal. The purpose of thimerosal, a preservative containing ethylmercury, was to prevent the contamination of vaccines by bacteria and fungi. Preservatives were needed because vaccines were often kept in multidose vials. Because the same vial was used to vaccinate more than one person, a needle to withdraw the vaccine could be inserted into the vial many times, increasing the risk of contamination. Children given the last few doses of a vaccine were at greatest risk. For example, in 1916, sixty-eight children developed severe systemic infections, twenty-six developed local abscesses, and four died after receipt of a multidose typhoid vaccine contaminated with the bacterium *Staphylococcus*. As a consequence of this and similar incidents, preservatives like thimerosal have been required for vaccines since the 1930s.

Despite its benefits, thimerosal was removed from most vaccines in the spring of 2001. The removal was precipitated by the contention that the levels of mercury in vaccines exceeded those recommended by the Environmental Protection Agency. (High levels of mercury can damage the nervous system.) Although these levels didn't exceed guidelines recommended by the Food and Drug Administration, the World Health Organization, or the Agency for Toxic Substances Disease Registry, thimerosal was removed as a precautionary measure. Not surprisingly, some parents felt that thimerosal had been removed because it caused neurological damage. So they sued the vaccine makers. But scientific evidence didn't support the notion that thimerosal was harmful. EPA guidelines were recommended for *methylmercury,* the kind of mercury found in the environment (such as in fish), not *ethylmercury,* the kind found in vaccines. Ethylmercury and methylmercury are very different. Ethylmercury is excreted from the body far more quickly than methylmercury and is therefore much less likely to accumulate. (An analogy can be made to the difference between ethylalcohol, the kind of alcohol contained in wine and beer, and methylalcohol, the kind contained in wood alcohol. Wood alcohol causes blindness; wine and beer don't.) Further, five large studies performed in Denmark, the United States, and the United Kingdom showed that children who received vaccines containing thimerosal were not more likely to have neurological problems—such as speech and language delays, tics, learning disabilities, or autism—than those who didn't receive these vaccines. In 2004 a group of scientists from the Institute of Medicine—an independent research organization within the National Academy of Sciences—reviewed studies that examined the relationship between thimerosal and neurologic damage. All the studies found the same thing: thimerosal, at the level contained in vaccines, didn't cause harm.

Although the science was against them, lawyers pressed forward;

to gain clients, they advertised on local radio and television stations for people who believed that their children had been hurt by thimerosal. Charles Lawrence, a lawyer from Hattiesburg, Mississippi, sent out questionnaires asking parents whether they had noticed any of the following after their children had received vaccines: irritability, confusion, insomnia, shyness, clumsiness, lack of coordination, mood swings, indifference, temper tantrums, toe walking, agitation, a desire to be alone, or an increased tendency to masturbate. If they had, said Mr. Lawrence, they could claim that thimerosal in the vaccine was the cause. Mr. Lawrence attached a form for parents to sign granting him 40 percent of the total recovery (50 percent if the verdict was appealed). About three hundred separate lawsuits against vaccine makers are pending in U.S. courts, and vaccine makers have already spent more than $400 million in their defense. The first lawsuits were scheduled to go to court in March 2007. Vaccine makers are bracing for the possibility of awards that could threaten their capacity to remain in the vaccine business.

Another problem with the federal vaccine compensation program can be found in the stories of two teenagers. In 2001 a thirteen-year-old boy was traveling to Tampa, Florida, with his parents. Before getting into the car to go to the airport, he fainted. The mother, assuming that her son had tripped, continued the journey, but when they got to the airport, the boy fainted again. Just before the second attack the child seemed to be disoriented and confused. The mother quickly called one of the gate attendants, who called the airport doctor. By the time the doctor arrived, the child was alert and attentive. A blood test later revealed the boy's diagnosis. The second boy was sixteen years old. In 2002, while walking to school, he noticed that his left leg hurt. At the hospital, his left knee was found to be hot, red, tender, and swollen. To make a diagnosis, the doctor put a needle into the knee, withdrew fluid, and sent the fluid for laboratory tests. Typically the knee has small quantities of fluid that contain few, if any, white blood cells. But the boy's knee contained large quantities of fluid and 197,000 white blood cells. Again a blood test revealed the diagnosis.

Although these boys had very different symptoms, they had the same ailment: Lyme disease, caused by the bacterium *Borrelia burgdorferi*. Lyme bacteria, which enter the bloodstream by the bite of a

tick, can infect either the joints (and cause arthritis) or the lining of the
heart, causing disruption of electrical impulses necessary for the heart
to beat. The first boy fainted because—for a few seconds—his heart had
stopped beating. The second boy was progressively less able to run,
walk, or stand. About twenty-three thousand people in the United
States are affected by Lyme disease every year.

During the course of these illnesses, the parents of both children
asked the same question: Why was there no vaccine to prevent Lyme
disease? Ironically there was: in December 1998 the Food and Drug
Administration had licensed a Lyme vaccine. The vaccine was made
using a protein located on the surface of the bacteria. Within months of
the release of the vaccine, some people complained of chronic arthritis
and sued the vaccine maker, GlaxoSmithKline.

Given the biology of Lyme disease and Lyme vaccine, it didn't
make sense that the vaccine would cause chronic arthritis. During
natural infection, Lyme bacteria enter the joints, multiply, and cause
intense inflammation. The Lyme vaccine, consisting of only one bacterial protein, doesn't enter the joints, doesn't reproduce itself, and
doesn't cause joint inflammation. Two large studies confirmed the
biological implausibility that the Lyme vaccine caused chronic arthritis. Either Lyme vaccine or no vaccine was given to twenty thousand
people, who were observed for two years. The incidence of chronic
arthritis—a fairly common disease in older adults—was the same in
both groups. But lawyers filed many lawsuits on behalf of people
claming that the Lyme vaccine had caused them to suffer chronic arthritis, as well as muscle pain, headaches, forgetfulness, memory loss,
paralysis, and fatigue. GlaxoSmithKline spent millions of dollars defending its product. The media reported that Lyme vaccine might
cause chronic arthritis and sales decreased. In 2002 the vaccine was
taken off the market. Now people who live in areas where Lyme disease is prevalent can only hope that they are not among those who are
permanently and severely harmed by the bacteria.

Usually when a vaccine is licensed and recommended, it is covered
by the federal compensation program. Unfortunately not all vaccines
are covered—only those recommended for *routine* use in children.
Because the Lyme vaccine wasn't recommended for all adolescents
(unlike most infectious diseases, Lyme disease doesn't occur in all

areas of the United States), it wasn't covered. So the vaccine was left to survive the abuses of personal injury lawyers and the inaccurate media reports that inevitably follow. As a consequence, a vaccine that worked and was safe is no longer available. Because of fears of litigation, it is unlikely that a second Lyme vaccine will ever be made.

Another problem with the federal vaccine compensation program is that it does not include an unborn child when the mother is immunized. Newborns are occasionally infected by a bacterium called group B streptococcus (GBS). GBS infects the bloodstream, the brain, and the spinal cord; every year in the United States about two thousand babies are infected with GBS and one hundred die. GBS kills more children in the first month of life than any other bacterial infection. Unfortunately, most vaccines in the United States and the world aren't given until a baby reaches one or two months—too late to prevent GBS.

In 1988 Carol Baker, a pediatrician and researcher at Baylor University in Houston, Texas, found a way to eliminate GBS infections in babies by immunizing pregnant women with a GBS vaccine. She found that her vaccine induced protective levels of GBS antibodies in the mother's blood and that these protective antibodies were passed on to the baby before birth. Although several pharmaceutical companies were interested in Dr. Baker's findings, none stepped forward to develop her vaccine because they didn't dare immunize pregnant women. Pharmaceutical companies know that about 2 percent of all children born in the United States have birth defects and that, by chance alone, if one hundred mothers were immunized with a GBS vaccine, two would bear children with birth defects. Even if study after study showed that the incidence of birth defects was the same in women who got the vaccine as in women who didn't, manufacturers couldn't trust that such studies would be appreciated by judges and juries. So a technology that would clearly save lives sits on the shelf. "We could make a group B strep vaccine tomorrow," said one senior pharmaceutical company scientist. "But it would have to be given to pregnant women and we couldn't handle the liability."

In 2004 a one-month-old boy infected with GBS was admitted to a hospital in northern New Jersey. GBS had infected the child's brain and spinal cord; as a consequence, it is unlikely that he will ever see, hear, or walk. The boy's parents, devastated by the severity of their son's illness and confusing a bad outcome with bad care, were angry and wanted to sue the hospital. Their immediate instinct to sue in part explains why we don't have a GBS vaccine that could have prevented the problem.

Finally, in addition to weaknesses in the federal compensation program, liability insurance has dramatically increased the cost of making all medical products and, as a consequence, companies have slowly abandoned lower-revenue products like vaccines. In 2003 two of the remaining four vaccine makers reduced their research and development budgets for vaccine. "The numbers for pediatric vaccines just don't add up any more," said a senior pharmaceutical company executive. "When you compare vaccines to other products, they fall below the line—well below the line." Companies now spend more money developing products that will be used every day and that will make large profits (such as drugs for obesity, high cholesterol, Alzheimer's disease, diabetes, impotency, and hair loss) than for products that would be used once in a lifetime and make small profits (such as vaccines and antibiotics). For example, a one-year supply of Lipitor, a cholesterol-lowering agent, costs about $1,600; a one-year supply of influenza vaccine costs about $8.00. It is, therefore, not surprising that annual sales for Lipitor are greater than the entire worldwide revenues for all vaccines. For the four companies that still make vaccines, gross annual revenues from vaccines are less than 10 percent of total revenues; internationally vaccines account for about 1.5 percent of total revenues. Pharmaceutical companies are businesses, not public health agencies; they could stop making vaccines tomorrow without much of an impact on their bottom line.

So what is the solution? One solution would be to pay more for vaccines. The federal government buys about 55–60 percent of all vaccines used in the United States through the Vaccines for Children (VFC) Program. The purpose of the program, started in 1994, was to make sure that all uninsured or underinsured children would get the vaccines that they needed. The program resulted in an increase in the number of children in the United States that were vaccinated. But the federal government, as a large single purchaser of vaccines, inadvertently created a functional cap on vaccine prices and dramatically shrunk the private market. To encourage pharmaceutical companies to continue to make vaccines, Congress would have to pay more money for existing and new vaccines through the VFC program. People would have to place a higher value on preventive medicine and lobby their representatives in Congress to do the same—something that is unlikely to happen soon.

Another solution would be to reduce the cost of making vaccines without lowering standards of vaccine quality. This wouldn't be hard to do. Costs could be lowered by ensuring that compensation for harm caused by vaccines came only through the federal vaccine compensation program, that all vaccines were part of the program, and that all those affected by vaccines, such as the unborn child of a pregnant woman, were covered; money saved by making these changes would not be money spent making products better or safer. Because the vaccine injury compensation program would be the final arbiter on all questions of vaccine safety, claims judged to be without merit would be dismissed, and claimants would not have the option to sue pharmaceutical companies on their own. For this solution to work, we would have to change our attitudes about lawsuits.

We sue pharmaceutical companies because we want them to pay for our health care and because we want to punish them. In the United States we believe that injury deserves compensation and that serious injury deserves serious compensation. Phen-phen—a weight-loss product developed by Wyeth—was found to be a rare cause of heart disease only after it had been used by millions of people. As a consequence, Wyeth will pay about $16 billion in awards. In the aftermath of the phen-phen settlement, Wyeth, like many pharmaceutical companies, has been driven even further away from small-market products like vaccines. To ensure that life-saving products continue to be made, we would have to resist the lure of a court system that functions as a national lottery for health care—because the courts are a terrible place to assure health care. For example, in 2004 personal injury lawyers in Philadelphia sued several doctors for negligence; they asked for $40 million in damages. During the trial, defense lawyers made it clear that they were willing to settle for $17 million. The plantiff (i.e., the patient) thought he could do better, so he continued with the trial. When it was over, the jury handed down its verdict—for the defense. The patient got nothing. During the trial the patient had variously faced the possibilities of receiving $40 million, $17 million, or nothing. The crapshoot of court verdicts is a wildly inefficient and ineffective way to determine whether and at what level someone should receive health care.

Also, punitive lawsuits, by increasing the cost of liability insurance, have dramatically increased the cost of making medical products and have made products like vaccines less attractive. In the end, we have to ask ourselves who is being punished by such lawsuits. If children are hurt by a vaccine, they will have no trouble finding someone to represent their interests. Personal injury lawyers will line up to be the chosen representatives, and the media will gladly tell their stories across the country. But who will represent the interests of the thousands of children hospitalized, permanently harmed, and killed by viruses and bacteria for which existing vaccines are in short supply or for which new vaccines may never be developed?

Epilogue

Take one moment to embrace those gentle heroes we left behind.
—Michael O'Donnell

THE CUTTER INCIDENT CAUSED AN IMMEDIATE change in the way that vaccines were made and regulated in the United States. As a consequence, companies made a safer polio vaccine and children's lives were saved. But the price paid for this knowledge was that many children were paralyzed for the rest of their lives. On the wall of the Vietnam Veterans Memorial in Washington, D.C., are inscribed the words of Major Michael O'Donnell, killed in action on February 7, 1978: "And in time when men reflect and feel safe to call that war insane, take one moment to embrace those gentle heroes we left behind." The fight against diseases that kill our children is, in a way, like a war. When we fight back, innocent people are sometimes wrongly hurt. Although medical tragedies may be inevitable, they are nonetheless never acceptable.

Anne Gottsdanker was among hundreds of gentle souls left behind in the war against polio. After taking courses in Paris and England during high school, Anne graduated from Reed College in Portland, Oregon, became a biology teacher, received a master's degree in elementary education from the University of California, Santa Barbara, and began a career as an English instructor at Arizona State University. In 1979, at the age of thirty, she met her husband, Michael, and, after a one-month engagement, was married in her parents' backyard. In May 1983 Anne delivered her first daughter, Melanie Leela, and in July 1988 she delivered her second, Elizabeth Michelle. Today, Anne teaches reading at Antelope Valley Community College and continues to travel to Europe, now with her daughters.

But Anne Gottsdanker is still bound by the tragedy that occurred at Cutter Laboratories. Her legs remain severely paralyzed, she cannot walk without the support of crutches, and she wears a large brace because of repeated dislocations of her knee. She dreads the day when she will be permanently bound to a wheelchair. "I wish the Cutters could see me now," she says quietly. "See how hard it is to live like this. I've worked hard, but when you have a disability that people can see, they're a lot less accepting—that never changes."

Anne's daughter Melanie is now twenty-two years old; her younger daughter, Elizabeth, is seventeen. It is likely that soon both will have children of their own. In part because of the verdict in *Gottsdanker v. Cutter Laboratories,* Anne's grandchildren might have to face diseases for which no vaccines will be developed—diseases like group A streptococcus, which causes rheumatic fever and severe skin infections; cytomegalovirus, which causes mental retardation, impaired vision, hearing loss, and cerebral palsy; adenovirus, respiratory syncytial virus, and parainfluenza virus, which cause pneumonia; and enteroviruses, herpesviruses, and arboviruses (like West Nile virus), which cause meningitis. All of these infections routinely cause children in the United States and in the world to be hospitalized and to die. Although the technology is available to prevent much of this suffering, the infrastructure and desire necessary to develop these vaccines are fading. Ironically, in an attempt to protect children from harm, we have inadvertently exposed them to a greater harm.

Notes

Prologue

Page

xi American lifespan: J. P. Bunker, H. S. Frazier, and F. Mosteller, Improving health: Measuring effects of medical care, *Milbank Quarterly* 72 (1994): 225–58.

xi Before vaccines: Plotkin and Orenstein, *Vaccines.*

xi Smallpox: M. Radetsky, Smallpox: A history of its rise and fall, *Pediatric Infectious Disease Journal* 18 (1999): 85–93.

xi Vaccine shortages: J. Cohen, U.S. vaccine supply falls seriously short, *Science* 295 (2002): 1998–2001; National Vaccine Advisory Committee, Strengthening the supply of routinely recommended vaccines in the United States: Recommendations of the National Vaccine Advisory Committee, *Journal of the American Medical Association* 290 (2003): 3122–28.

xii Influenza epidemic: Data presented to the Advisory Committee for Immunization Practices, Centers for Disease Control and Prevention, June 23, 2004.

Introduction

The story of Anne Gottsdanker and quotes from Josephine Gottsdanker were found in the reporter's transcript, *Gottsdanker v. Cutter Laboratories,* District Court of Appeal of the State of California, First Appellate District, 1 Civ. 18,413 and 18,414.

1 Pittsburgh nurse: Cited in Carter, *Breakthrough,* 107.

2 Phoenix mother: Cited in Black, *Shadow of Polio,* 15.

3 Former camper: Interview with Irv Gomprecht, Baltimore, MD, February 23, 2003.

3 Anne Gottsdanker's recollection of disease: Interview with Anne Gottsdanker, June 12, 2000.

Chapter 1: Little White Coffins

The two best sources for information about the 1916 polio epidemic in New York City are Emerson, *Monograph,* and Rogers, *Dirt and Disease;* all statements by New York City health commissioner Haven Emerson were obtained from the Emerson monograph. Excellent descriptions of John Kolmer, Maurice Brodie, and their ill-fated vaccines can be found in the following: Berg, *Polio,* 50–59; Carter, *Breakthrough,* 20–24; Gould, *Summer Plague,* 66–69; Klein, *Trial,* 20–23; Paul, *Poliomyelitis,* 252–62; Rogers, *Dirt and Disease,* 171–72; Smith, *Patenting the Sun,* 72; Williams, *Virus Hunters,* 273–78.

4 Social worker regarding hearses: Cited in Al Burns, "The Scourge of 1916 . . . America's First and Worst Polio Epidemic," *American Legion Magazine,* September 1966, 45.

4 New York City epidemic: Berg, *Polio,* 1–7; Carter, *Breakthrough,* 8–11; Gould, *Summer Plague,* 3–28; Klein, *Trial,* 3–9; Paul, *Poliomyelitis,* 148–60; Smith, *Patenting the Sun,* 31–37; Williams, *Virus Hunters,* 239–40; Wilson, *Margin,* 36–40; Al Burns, "The Scourge of 1916 . . . America's First and Worst Polio Epidemic," *American Legion Magazine,* September 1966; "All United to Check Infantile Paralysis," *New York Times,* June 30, 1916; "Day Shows 12 Dead by Infant Paralysis," *New York Times,* July 2, 1916; "Bar All Children from the Movies in Paralysis War," *New York Times,* July 4, 1916; "Infantile Paralysis a Scourge and Puzzle," *New York Times,* July 9, 1916; "Believes Paralysis a Throat Infection: Dr. Bryant Says Germs Attack Only Membranes in the Air Passages of Head," *New York Times,* July 10, 1916; "31 Die of Paralysis; 162 More Ill in City," *New York Times,* July 15, 1916; "Suggests Serum for All Children: Dr. Zinghar Thinks Paralysis Might Be Checked by Using It as Preventive," *New York Times,* August 15, 1916; "Fears Subway Flies Help Spread Plague: Edward Hatch, Jr., Asserts That Millions Breed in Refuse Left in Excavations," *New York Times,* August 18, 1916; "Drop in Paralysis Encourages City: Daily Average of New Cases in New York Falls from 173 to 131," *New York Times,* August 18, 1916; "Doctors at Odds about Paralysis; Sheffield Advises and Lovett Opposes Use of Strychnine and Massage; Adrenaline Is Recommended," *New York Times,* August 20, 1916; "Oyster Bay Revolts over Poliomyelitis," *New York Times,* August 29, 1916; "Paralysis Defers College Openings," *New York Times,* August 31, 1916; "Meltzer Assails Auto-Inoculation; Rockefeller Institute Scientist Would Forbid Its Use in Paralysis Cases; Serum from Horse Blood; Physicians in this City See Value in Its Administration—Chickens Blamed for Epidemic," *New York Times,* September 2, 1916; "Let Children Romp as Epidemic Wanes," *New York Times,* September 5, 1916; "Believes Mosquito Spreads Paralysis: Dr. C. S. Braddock, Jr., Asserts That Careful Observations Support Theory," *New York Times,* September 9, 1916.

4 Previous polio epidemics in the United States: Emerson, *Monograph,* table 1.

5 Social worker regarding babies: Cited in Al Burns, "The Scourge of 1916 . . . America's First and Worst Polio Epidemic," *American Legion Magazine*, September 1966, 45.

5 Mrs. Dasnoit: Berg, *Polio*, 4.

6 Anna Henry: "Death Note for Nurse Reporting Plague Cases," *New York Times*, July 23, 1916.

8 Dr. Robert Guilfoy: Al Burns, "The Scourge of 1916 . . . America's First and Worst Polio Epidemic," *American Legion Magazine*, September 1966, 47.

8 New York City residents' panic: Ibid., 45.

9 Wood shavings and "Sol": Berg, *Polio*, 5.

9 Retan: Wilson, *Margin*, 45.

9 Last three weeks of August 1916: Emerson, *Monograph*.

9 Percentage of deaths: Al Burns, "The Scourge of 1916 . . . America's First and Worst Polio Epidemic," *American Legion Magazine*, September 1966.

9 Influenza deaths: "The American Experience: Influenza 1918"; http://www.pbs .org/wgbh/amex/influenza/tguide/index.html.

9 American war deaths: American War Library; http://members.aol.com/ usregistry/allwars.htm.

10 World's knowledge of polio: Al Burns, "The Scourge of 1916 . . . America's First and Worst Polio Epidemic," *American Legion Magazine*, September 1966, 15.

10 Causes of polio: Emerson, *Monograph*, 75–77.

10 Landsteiner: Paul, *Poliomyelitis*, 98–106; Berg, *Polio*, 11.

10 Kling: Paul, *Poliomyelitis*, 126–36; Berg, *Polio*, 14.

11 Flexner: Paul, *Poliomyelitis*, 107–25; Berg, *Polio*, 50.

11 Hopkins researchers: Howe and Bodian, *Neural Mechanisms;* D. Bodian: Experimental studies on passive immunization against poliomyelitis, I: Protection with human gamma globulin against intramuscular inoculation and combined passive and active immunization, *American Journal of Hygiene* 54 (1951): 132–43; Viremia in experimental poliomyelitis, I: General aspects of infection after intravascular inoculation with strains of high and low invasiveness, *American Journal of Hygiene* 60 (1954): 339–57; D. Bodian and R. S. Paffenbarger, Poliomyelitis infections in households: Frequency of viremia and specific antibody response, *American Journal of Hygiene* 60 (1954): 83–98; H. A. Howe, Antibody response of chimpanzees and human beings to formalin-inactivated trivalent poliomyelitis vaccine, *American Journal of Hygiene* 56 (1952): 265–86; Poliomyelitis infection in immunized chimpanzees, *Annals of the New York Academy of Science*, 1954, 1014–21; Studies of active immunogenesis in poliomyelitis, I: Persistence and recall of homotypic and heterotypic superinfection of neutralization antibody originally induced in chimpanzees by vaccination or infection, *American Journal of Hygiene* 60 (1954): 371–91; Studies of active immunogenesis in poliomyelitis, II: Lack of immunity in chimpanzees

receiving formol-inactivated vaccines of marginal antigenic potency, *American Journal of Hygiene* 60 (1954): 392–95; H. A. Howe, D. Bodian, and I. M. Morgan, Subclinical poliomyelitis in the chimpanzee and its relation to alimentary reinfection, *American Journal of Hygiene* 51 (1950): 85–108; I. M. Morgan, Level of serum antibody associated with intracerebral immunity in monkeys vaccinated with Lansing poliomyelitis virus, *Journal of Immunology* 62 (1949): 301–10.

12 Jenner and smallpox vaccine: B. Moss, Vaccinia virus: A tool for research and vaccine development, *Science* 252 (1991): 1662–67; M. Radetsky, Smallpox: A history of its rise and fall, *Pediatric Infectious Disease Journal* 18 (1999): 85–93; P. Radetsky, *Invaders*, 25–37.

13 Pasteur and rabies vaccine: P. Radetsky, *Invaders*, 51–58.

14 Theiler and yellow fever vaccine: Williams, *Virus Hunters*, 154–75.

14 Kolmer description: Paul, *Poliomyelitis*, 256.

15 Coolidge: Cited in http://calvincoolidge.us/pages/1/ page1.html; http://www.theatlantic.com/unbound/polypro/pp2003-12-31.htm.

15 Kolmer scientific studies: J. A. Kolmer: Active immunization against acute anterior poliomyelitis with ricinolated vaccine, *Journal of Immunology* 32 (1937): 341–56; Antibody in relation to immunity in acute poliomyelitis, *Journal of Immunology* 31 (1936): 119–34; An improved method of preparing the Kolmer poliomyelitis vaccine, *American Journal of Public Health* 26 (1936): 149–57; Infection, susceptibility, and vaccination in acute anterior poliomyelitis, *Journal of the Medical Society of New Jersey* 32 (1935): 491–93; Susceptibility and immunity in relation to vaccination with acute anterior poliomyelitis, *Journal of the American Medical Association* 105 (1935): 1956–62; Vaccination against acute anterior poliomyelitis, *American Journal of Public Health* 26 (1936): 126–35; J. A. Kolmer and A. M. Rule, Concerning vaccination of monkeys against acute anterior poliomyelitis, *Journal of Immunology* 26 (1934): 505–15; A successful method for vaccination against acute anterior poliomyelitis virus, *American Journal of Medical Science* 188 (1934): 510–14; J. A. Kolmer, G. F. Klugh, and A. M. Rule, A successful method for vaccination against acute anterior poliomyelitis, *Journal of the American Medical Association* 104 (1935): 456–60.

16 Brodie description: Paul, *Poliomyelitis*, 256–62; Benison, *Rivers*, 183–85.

16 Brodie studies: Berg, *Polio*, 53–55; M. Brodie, Active immunization in monkeys against poliomyelitis with germicidally inactivated virus, *Journal of Immunology* 28 (1934): 1–18; Active immunization in monkeys against poliomyelitis with germicidally inactivated virus, *Science* 79 (1934): 594–95; Active immunization of children against poliomyelitis with formalin-inactivated virus suspension, *Proceedings of the Society of Experimental Biology and Medicine* 32 (1934): 300–302; Active immunization of children against poliomyelitis with formalin-inactivated virus suspension, *New York Academy of Medicine*, 1934, 30–32; M. Brodie and W. H. Park, Active immunization against poliomyelitis, *New*

York State Journal of Medicine, 1935, 815–18; Active immunization against poliomyelitis, *Journal of the American Medical Association* 105 (1935): 1089–92; Active immunization against poliomyelitis, *American Journal of Public Health* 26 (1936): 119–25.

16 Brodie regarding perfect safety: M. Brodie, Active immunization of children against poliomyelitis with formalin-inactivated virus suspension, *Proceedings of the Society of Experimental Biology and Medicine* 32 (1934): 300–302.

16 Description of Rivers: Smith, *Patenting the Sun,* 113.

16 Children killed by Kolmer's vaccine: Letters from city health departments describing cases of polio following Kolmer's vaccine, Thomas Rivers Archive, American Philosophical Society, Philadelphia, PA.

17 Comments by Kolmer and results of St. Louis meeting: Benison, *Rivers,* 184–90.

17 Comments by Leake, Rivers, and Kolmer: Cited in ibid.

18 Brodie's vaccine questioned by Leake: J. P. Leake, Poliomyelitis following vaccination against the disease, *Journal of the American Medical Association* 105 (1935): 2152.

18 Brodie's death: Williams, *Virus Hunters,* 278.

Chapter 2: Back to the Drawing Board

Excellent discussions of FDR, O'Connor, and the March of Dimes can be found in Berg, *Polio;* Carter, *Breakthrough* and *Gentle Legions;* Gould, *Summer Plague;* Klein, *Trial;* Rogers, *Dirt and Disease;* Smith, *Patenting the Sun;* Williams, *Virus Hunters;* and Wilson, *Margin.*

19 Description of FDR by Churchill: Goodwin, *No Ordinary Time,* 606.

19 Description of FDR's physical activities and attempts to walk: Ibid., 16.

20 Skinny, frostbitten newsboy: Carter, *Breakthrough,* 12.

20 "To dance so that others may walk": Carter, *Breakthrough,* 14.

20 FDR birthday broadcast: Ibid.

21 De Kruif background: Benison, *Rivers,* 180.

21 De Kruif against doctors: "Our Medicine Men, by One of Them," *The Century,* 1922.

21 Flexner fires de Kruif and waspish pen: Gould, *Summer Plague,* 80.

21 *Arrowsmith:* S. Lewis, *Arrowsmith* (New York: Harcourt, Brace, and World, 1925).

22 *Microbe Hunters:* P. de Kruif, *Microbe Hunters* (New York: Harcourt, Brace, and World, 1926).

22 De Kruif regarding cripples: De Kruif, *Sweeping Wind,* 177.

22 De Kruif regarding nasal spray therapy: Gould, *Summer Plague,* 69.

22 Nasal spray studies: C. A. Armstrong, Prevention of intravenously inoculated poliomyelitis of monkeys by intranasal instillation of picric acid, *Public Health Reports* 51 (1936): 241–43; Experience with the picric acid-alum spray in the prevention of poliomyelitis in Alabama, 1936, *American Journal of Public Health* 27 (1937): 103–11; M. M. Peet, D. H. Echols, and H. J. Richter, The chemical prophylaxis for poliomyelitis, *Journal of the American Medical Association* 108 (1937): 2184–87; E. W. Schultz, Prevention of intranasally inoculated poliomyelitis in monkeys by previous intranasal irrigation with chemical agents, *Proceedings of the Society of Experimental Medicine and Biology* 34 (1936): 133–35; Immunity and prophylaxis in poliomyelitis, *Journal of the American Medical Association* 107 (1936): 2102–04; E. W. Schultz, and L. P. Gebhardt, Zinc sulfate prophylaxis in poliomyelitis, *Journal of the American Medical Association* 108 (1937): 2182–84.

22 Roosevelt announces new foundation: Carter, *Breakthrough*, 15.

24 Production of a good vaccine: Ibid., 25.

24 Burnet and Macnamara: Paul, *Poliomyelitis*, 225–31.

25 Polio virus typing: Excellent descriptions of the polio virus typing programs can be found in Berg, *Polio;* Carter, *Breakthrough;* Gould, *Summer Plague;* Klein, *Trial;* Rogers, *Dirt and Disease;* Smith, *Patenting the Sun;* Williams, *Virus Hunters;* and Wilson, *Margin.*

26 Rabies vaccine and paralysis: S. A. Plotkin, C. E. Rupprecht, and H. Koprowski, Rabies vaccine, in Plotkin and Orenstein, *Vaccines,* 1025–26.

26 Enders background: Smith, *Patenting the Sun,* 125–26.

26 Enders, Weller, and Robbins studies: Weller, *Growing Pathogens,* 75–90; J. F. Enders, T. H. Weller, and F. C. Robbins, Cultivation of the Lansing strain of poliomyelitis virus in cultures of various human tissues, *Science* 109 (1949): 85–87; T. H. Weller, F. C. Robbins, and J. F. Enders, Cultivation of poliomyelitis virus in cultures of human foreskin and embryonic tissues, *Proceedings of the Society of Experimental Biology and Medicine* 72 (1949): 153–55; F. C. Robbins, J. F. Enders, and T. H. Weller, Cytopathogenic effect of poliomyelitis virus in vitro on human embryonic tissues, *Proceedings of the Society of Experimental Biology and Medicine* 75 (1950): 370–74.

27 Robbins on experiments and winning the Nobel Prize: Interview with Frederick Robbins, July 29, 1998.

28 O'Connor on Salk: Cited in Gould, *Summer Plague,* 129.

28 Jonas Salk background: Excellent discussions of Salk's personal life and early medical and research career can be found in Berg, *Polio;* Carter, *Breakthrough;* Gould, *Summer Plague;* Klein, *Trial;* Rogers, *Dirt and Disease,* Smith, *Patenting the Sun;* Williams, *Virus Hunters;* and Wilson, *Margin.*

30 Donna Salk on Jonas: Interview with Donna Salk, February 10, 1999.

30 Youngner on hard work: Interview with Julius Youngner, July 14, 1998.

31 Weaver on Salk: Cited in Carter, *Breakthrough*, 68–69.

31 "Damned industrial plant": Carter, *Breakthrough*, 4.

32 Salk polio experiments: Interview with Darrell Salk, son of Jonas Salk, February 14, 2004; J. E. Salk, Principles of immunization as applied to poliomyelitis and influenza, *American Journal of Public Health* 43 (1953): 1384–98; Recent studies on immunization against poliomyelitis, *Pediatrics* 12 (1953): 471–82; Studies in human subjects on active immunization against poliomyelitis, *Journal of the American Medical Association* 151 (1953): 1081–98; Vaccination against paralytic poliomyelitis: Performance and prospects, *American Journal of Public Health* 45 (1955): 575–96; Considerations in the preparation and use of poliomyelitis virus vaccine, *Journal of the American Medical Association* 158 (1955): 1239–48; J. E. Salk, and J. B. Gori, A review of theoretical, experimental, and practical considerations in the use of formaldehyde for the inactivation of poliovirus, *Annals of the New York Academy of Sciences* 83 (1959): 609–37; J. E. Salk, U. Krech, J. S. Youngner, B. L. Bennett, L. J. Lewis, and P. L. Bazeley, Formaldehyde treatment and safety testing of experimental poliomyelitis vaccine, *American Journal of Public Health* 44 (1954): 563–70; J. Salk and D. Salk, Control of influenza and poliomyelitis with killed virus vaccines, *Science* 195 (1977): 834–47.

34 Mahoney virus: D. Bodian, Viremia in experimental poliomyelitis, I: General aspects of infection after intravascular inoculation with strains of high and low invasiveness, *American Journal of Hygiene* 60 (1954): 339–57.

34 Salk chooses Mahoney because of virulence: Discussion with Neal Nathanson, former director of the Poliomyelitis Surveillance Unit, September 20, 2004.

34 Dangerous virus: Albert Sabin, testifying at hearings before the Committee on Interstate and Foreign Commerce, House of Representatives, Eighty-Fourth Congress, First Session, May 27, 1955.

35 Watson home: Smith, *Patenting the Sun*, 140–41.

35 Cochran on Salk: Cited in Carter, *Breakthrough*, 139.

36 Willowbrook: S. Krugman and R. Ward, Clinical and experimental studies of infectious hepatitis, *Pediatrics* 22 (1958): 1016–22; S. Krugman, The Willowbrook hepatitis studies revisited: Ethical aspects, *Reviews of Infectious Diseases* 8 (1986): 157–62.

38 Salk's reactions to Watson and Polk studies: Carter, *Breakthrough*, 141–53.

38 Smadel pushes for vaccine: Paul, *Poliomyelitis*, 419.

38 Salk's radio broadcast: Carter, *Breakthrough*, 156–62.

39 Critic's response to radio broadcast: Carter, *Breakthrough*, 158.

39 Donna Salk on the immunization of her children: Interview with Donna Salk, February 10, 1999.

39 Joseph Bell: Benison, *Rivers*, 508–9.

40 Flicker of light: Carter, *Breakthrough*, 146.

42 Milzer's experiments: A. Milzer, S. O. Levinson, H. J. Shaughnessy et al., Immunogenicity studies in human subjects of trivalent tissue culture poliomyelitis vaccine inactivated by ultraviolet irradiation, *American Journal of Public Health* 44 (1954): 26–33.

43 Milzer on the limitations of Salk's method: Cited in W. L. Laurence, "Anti-Polio Vaccine Defended as Safe," *New York Times,* November 11, 1953. Salk to friend: Smith, *Patenting the Sun,* 243.

43 Gard: *Poliomyelitis: Papers and Discussions Presented at the Third International Poliomyelitis Conference* (Philadelphia and Montreal: Lippincott, 1955), 202–6; interview with Erling Norrby, polio researcher and former student of Sven Gard, July 21, 1998.

Chapter 3: The Grand Experiment

Excellent discussions of the field trial of Jonas Salk's vaccine and the announcement of the results can be found in Benison, *Rivers;* Carter, *Breakthrough;* Gould, *Summer Plague;* Klein, *Trial;* Rogers, *Dirt and Disease;* Smith, *Patenting the Sun;* Williams, *Virus Hunters;* and Wilson, *Margin.*

44 Jonas Salk on human error: J. E. Salk, U. Krech, J. S. Youngner, B. L. Bennett, L. J. Lewis, and P. L. Bazeley, Formaldehyde treatment and safety testing of experimental poliomyelitis vaccine, *American Journal of Public Health* 44 (1954): 563–70.

44 Number of people afflicted with polio: Center for Disease Control, Poliomyelitis Surveillance Summary 1974–1976; issued October 1977.

45 Salk on Parke-Davis: Cited in Carter, *Breakthrough,* 184.

45 Parke-Davis on Salk: Carter, *Breakthrough,* 197.

46 Salk on details of inactivation: J. E. Salk, U. Krech, J. S. Youngner, B. L. Bennett, L. J. Lewis, and P. L. Bazeley, Formaldehyde treatment and safety testing of experimental poliomyelitis vaccine, *American Journal of Public Health* 44 (1954): 563–70.

47 Salk on baking a cake: Cited in Robert Coughlan, "Science Moves in on Viruses," *Life,* June 22, 1955.

47 Salk protocol: Specifications and minimal requirements for poliomyelitis vaccine aqueous (polyvalent) as developed by Dr. Jonas E. Salk, Virus Research Laboratory, University of Pittsburgh, Pittsburgh, Pennsylvania (To be used for field studies to be conducted during 1954 under the auspices of the National Foundation for Infantile Paralysis), February 1, 1954 (provided by Dr. Martha Lepow).

47 "Dirty word": Cited in Carter, *Breakthrough,* 216.

47 "Damned research project": Ibid.

48 Cutter mistake: March of Dimes Archive; Salk and Sabin Polio Vaccine Rec-

ords, 1848–1990; Series 3: Salk Vaccine; Cutter Laboratories; Letter from Ralph Houlihan to Jonas Salk, June 1, 1954.

48 Workman description: Interview with Ruth Kirchstein, former researcher in the Division of Biologic Standards and former director of the National Institute of General Medical Services within the National Institutes of Health, October 7, 1998. (The Laboratory of Biologics Control became the Division of Biologic Standards within several months of the Cutter Incident.)

49 Workman on vaccine safety: Cited in Carter, *Breakthrough*, 221.

49 Rivers on dangerous vaccine: Cited in Benison, *Rivers*, 533.

49 Winchell: Smith, *Patenting the Sun*, 256–57; Gabler, *Winchell*, 471–72; Walter Winchell, "Walter Winchell of New York," *Daily Mirror*, April 9 and 26, 1954; "County in Michigan Cancels Polio Test," *New York Times*, April 10, 1954.

51 Salk on placebo: Cited in Carter, *Breakthrough*, 191–92.

52 Randy Kerr: Cited in Smith, *Patenting the Sun*, 267.

52 1954 field trial results: Francis, *Evaluation of 1954 Field Trial*; T. D. Dublin, 1954 poliomyelitis vaccine field trial: Plan, field operations, and follow-up observations, *Journal of the American Medical Association* 158 (1955): 1258–65; T. Francis Jr., Evaluation of the 1954 poliomyelitis field trial: Further studies on results determining the effectiveness of poliomyelitis vaccine (Salk) in preventing paralytic poliomyelitis, *Journal of the American Medical Association* 158 (1955): 1266–70.

52 Francis on vaccine as cause of paralysis: Francis, *Evaluation of 1954 Field Trial*, 19.

54 Salk on Ann Arbor: Cited in Carter, *Breakthrough*, 269.

54 Gallup poll: Carter, *Gentle Legions*, 133.

54 Observer on complexity of trial: Cited in Williams, *Virus Hunters*, 311.

54 1954 field trial, setting and announcement: W. L. Laurence, "Salk Polio Vaccine Proves Success; Millions Will Be Immunized Soon; City Schools Begin Shots April 25," *New York Times*, April 13, 1955; "54,000 Physicians See Digest on TV," *New York Times*, April 13, 1955; "Fanfare Ushers Verdict on Tests," *New York Times*, April 13, 1955; "Text of the Statements on Dr. Salk's Vaccine Evaluation," *New York Times*, April 13, 1955; "Age of Salk's Aides Averages under 40," *New York Times*, April 13, 1955.

55 National Foundation member on theatrical atmosphere: Cited in Carter, *Breakthrough*, 258.

55 Associated Press newsman: Leonard Engel, "The Salk Vaccine: What Caused the Mess?" *Harper's Magazine*, August 1955, 30.

55 "It works": Seavey, Smith, and Wagner, *Paralyzing Fear*, 189; "It Works," *Time*, April 25, 1955.

56 War ended: Cited in Williams, *Virus Hunters*, 315.

56 Francis angry at Salk: Cited in Carter, *Breakthrough*, 281.

56 Rivers angry at Salk: Ibid.

57 Salk on *See It Now* and in Ann Arbor: Cited in ibid., 264–65.

57 Hollywood premiere article: "Fanfare Ushers Verdict on Tests," *New York Times*, April 13, 1955.

57 Salk not unscathed: Cited in Carter, *Breakthrough*, 269.

Chapter 4: How Does It Feel to Be a Killer of Children?

The best discussion of the timeline for licensure, release, and withdrawal of Cutter's vaccine can be found in the technical report written by Surgeon General Leonard A. Scheele to Oveta Culp Hobby, secretary of the Department of Health, Education, and Welfare: Leonard A. Scheele, *Public Health Service Technical Report on Salk Poliomyelitis Vaccine* (U.S. Department of Health, Education, and Welfare, June 1955); referred to below as Scheele, *Technical Report*. This report was generously provided to the author by Dr. Thomas Weller. Summaries of the technical report can also be found in D. Bodian, T. Francis Jr., C. Larson, J. E. Salk, R. E. Shope, J. E. Smadel, and J. A. Shannon, Interim report, Public Health Service Technical Committee on poliomyelitis vaccine, *Journal of the American Medical Association* 159 (1955): 1444–47, and Technical report on poliomyelitis vaccine, *Public Health Reports* 70 (1955): 738–51. The founding and development of Cutter Laboratories is best described in Morris, *Cutter Laboratories,* vols. 1 and 2; unless otherwise stated, all quotes from Cutter executives Robert Cutter, Ted Cutter, and Harry Lange were taken from this source.

58 Hobby, great day: Cited in Carter, *Breakthrough*, 282.

59 Biologics Control Act: Hilts, *Protecting America's Health,* 69–70; William Egan, "The Biologics Control Act of 1902 and the Regulation of Biologics: A Brief Reflection"; http://www.fda.gov/cber/summaries/cent092302WE.pdf; Dennis B. Worthen, "The Pharmaceutical Industry: 1902–1952"; http://www .aphanet.org/about/sequisept01.html; "A Short History of the National Institutes of Health, Office of NIH History"; http://history.nih.gov/exhibits/history/docs/page_03.html.

59 Laboratory of Biologics Control: Reporter's transcript, *Gottsdanker v. Cutter Laboratories,* District Court of Appeal of the State of California, First Appellate District, 1 Civ. 18,413 and 18,414, 1097–99; Scheele, *Technical Report,* appendices B3 and B5.

59 Former employee on lack of expertise at the Laboratory of Biologics Control: Interviews with Ruth Kirchstein, October 7, 1998, and April 20, 1999.

60 Differences between National Foundation and Laboratory of Biologics Control requirements: Salk protocol: Specifications and minimal requirements for poliomyelitis vaccine aqueous (polyvalent) as developed by Dr. Jonas E. Salk, Virus Research Laboratory, University of Pittsburgh, Pittsburgh, Pennsylvania (To be used for field studies to be conducted during 1954 under the auspices of

the National Foundation for Infantile Paralysis), February 1, 1954 (provided by Dr. Martha Lepow); Minimum Requirements: Poliomyelitis Vaccine, May 20, 1954, September 13, 1954, December 14, 1954, and April 12, 1955 (1st revision).

61 Right to make imperfect vaccine: Testimony of Milton Veldee, former head of Laboratory of Biologics Control; reporter's transcript, *Gottsdanker v. Cutter Laboratories*, District Court of Appeal of the State of California, First Appellate District, 1 Civ. 18,413 and 18,414, 1851–1897.

61 Workman meeting: Carter, *Breakthrough*, 281–82.

62 Shaughnessy on the licensing meeting: Reporter's transcript, *Gottsdanker v. Cutter Laboratories*, District Court of Appeal of the State of California, First Appellate District, 1 Civ. 18,413 and 18,414, 1611.

62 Bernice Eddy: For biographical data, see Ohern, *Profiles,* 151–59; Curriculum vitae of Bernice Eddy, History of Medicine Division, National Library of Medicine, Bethesda, MD.

62 Bernice Eddy and inoculation of monkeys: Interview of Bernice Eddy by Dr. Wyndham Miles, historian, National Institutes of Health, November 3, 1964; History of Medicine Division, National Library of Medicine, Bethesda, MD.

63 Bernice Eddy and finding of live polio virus in Cutter's vaccine: N. Wade, Division of Biologic Standards: Scientific management questioned, *Science* 175 (1972): 966–70; Congressional Record—Senate, December 8, 1971, 45391–98; interview of Bernice Eddy by Dr. Wyndham Miles, historian, National Institutes of Health, November 3, 1964; History of Medicine Division, National Library of Medicine, Bethesda, MD.

63 Bernice Eddy dialogue with colleague and feeling of pending disaster: Interview with Maurice Hilleman, former director of Virus and Cell Biology Research, Merck Institute for Therapeutic Research, January 19, 1998. Dr. Hilleman is director of the Merck Institute for Vaccinology.

63 Julius Youngner reactions to Ann Arbor announcement: Interviews with Julius Youngner, July 14, 1998; July 15, 1999; and August 28, 1999.

65 Julius Youngner dialogue with Houlihan and observations at Cutter Laboratories: Ibid.

65 Julius Youngner and feelings of personal responsibility: Ibid.

65 Release of vaccine: Scheele, *Technical Report.*

66 First reports of cases of paralysis: N. Nathanson and A. D. Langmuir, The Cutter Incident: Poliomyelitis following formaldehyde-inactivated poliovirus vaccination in the United States during the spring of 1955, I: Background, *American Journal of Hygiene* 78 (1963): 16–28; Steven M. Spencer, "Where Are We Now on Polio?" *Saturday Evening Post*, September 10, 1955; memo of Victor H. Haas to William H. Sebrell and James Shannon, April 28, 1955 (generously provided by Dr. Martha Lepow).

67 Meeting, April 26, 1955: Details of the meeting and statements by participants, including Langmuir and Haas, can be found in Carter, *Breakthrough*, 309–10.

67 Participant's recollection: Ibid.

68 Langmuir on Cutter vaccine: Ibid.

68 Langmuir and drastic action: Ibid.

68 Telephone conference, April 27, 1955: Transcript of telephone conference, Room 122, Building 1, National Institutes of Health, April 27, 1955 (provided by Dr. Martha Lepow).

70 Haas response to telephone conference: Transcripts of Public Health Service Meetings (NIH) and Actions: April 27 and 28, 1955; May 1–3, 5, 7–11, 15, 27, 1955 (provided by Dr. Martha Lepow).

70 Description of Scheele: Steven M. Spencer, "Where Are We Now on Polio?" *Saturday Evening Post,* September 10, 1955; United States Department of Health and Human Services, Leonard A. Scheele (1948–1956): http://www.sur geongeneral.gov/library/history/bioburney.htm.

75 Cutter Laboratories produces tainted intravenous solution: "Warning Is Issued on Spoiled Glucose," *New York Times,* April 28, 1948; "Doctors Here Warned of Contaminated Drug," *New York Times,* May 7, 1948.

75 Description of Robert Cutter: Interview with James Gault, attorney for Cutter Laboratories, February 11, 1999.

77 Description of Walter Ward: Interview with James Gault, February 11, 1999; interviews with Ward coworkers Frank Deromedi and Robert Routh, February 11, 1999; interviews with David L. Cutter, son of Robert Cutter and director of Cutter Laboratories from 1967 until its acquisition by Bayer AG in 1974, August 20, 1998, and February 11, 1999.

77 Cutter first on the market: Scheele, *Technical Report,* appendix A 8.

77 Telegrams from William Workman to Walter Ward and from Cutter Laboratories to customers: Provided by David L. Cutter.

78 Cutter press release: Letter from Robert K. Cutter to stockholders, May 1955 (provided by David L. Cutter).

79 Scheele press release: Cited in Williams, *Virus Hunters,* 328.

79 Scheele and Cutter responses: B. Furman, "One Firm's Vaccine Barred: 6 Polio Cases Are Studied," *New York Times,* April 28, 1955; M. Kaplan: "All Banned Cutter Vaccine Here Found," *New York Times,* April 29, 1955, and "300,000 Got Cutter Shots; City Tightens Rule on Sales," *New York Times,* April 30, 1955; "Experts on Polio Say Inoculations Should Continue," *New York Times,* May 1, 1955.

79 Salk reactions to Cutter Incident: Cited in Carter, *Breakthrough,* 315.

79 Donna Salk's recollection: Interview with Donna Salk, February 10, 1999.

80 Friend's recollections: Interview with Richard Carter, Salk biographer, November 25, 1998.

80 Weller reaction to Cutter Incident: Interviews with Thomas Weller, October 27, 1998; November 7, 1998; and December 28, 1998.

80 New York County Medical Society grievances: M. Kaplan "300,000 Got Cutter Shots; City Tightens Rule on Sales," *New York Times,* April 30, 1955.

80 Alton Ochsner: Williams, *Virus Hunters,* 329.

80 John Ochsner on loss of nephew: Interview with John Ochsner by Beth Waters, May 1999.

80 Tom Coleman: Interview with Thomas Coleman, former medical writer and public relations director for the Virus Research Laboratory at the University of Pittsburgh, July 21, 1999.

81 Robert Routh: Interview with Robert Routh, former employee of Cutter Laboratories responsible for polio vaccine manufacture, February 11, 2000.

81 Frank Deromedi: Interview with Frank Deromedi, former supervisor of polio vaccine manufacture for Cutter Laboratories, February 11, 2000.

82 David Cutter story: Interviews with David L. Cutter, August 20, 1998, and February 11, 1999.

Chapter 5: A Man-Made Polio Epidemic

The definitive discussions of the number of cases of paralysis and death caused by the Cutter vaccine can be found in Scheele, *Technical Report,* and the following three-part article: N. Nathanson and A. D. Langmuir, The Cutter Incident: Poliomyelitis following formaldehyde-inactivated poliovirus vaccination in the United States during the spring of 1955, I: Background, *American Journal of Hygiene* 78 (1963): 16–28; The Cutter Incident: Poliomyelitis following formaldehyde-inactivated poliovirus vaccination in the United States during the spring of 1955, II: Relationship of poliomyelitis to Cutter vaccine, *American Journal of Hygiene* 78 (1963): 29–60; The Cutter Incident: Poliomyelitis following formaldehyde-inactivated poliovirus vaccination in the United States during the spring of 1955, III: Comparison of the clinical character of vaccinated and contact cases occurring after use of high rate lots of Cutter vaccine, *American Journal of Hygiene* 78 (1963): 61–81. See also D. Bodian, T. Francis Jr., C. Larson, J. E. Salk, R. E. Shope, J. E. Smadel, and J. A. Shannon, Interim report, Public Health Service Technical Committee on poliomyelitis vaccine, *Journal of the American Medical Association* 159 (1955): 1444–47.

83 Salk terrible feeling: Cited in Williams, *Virus Hunters,* 329.

83 Susan Pierce: Steven M. Spencer, "Where Are We Now on Polio?" *Saturday Evening Post,* September 10, 1955; "Girl Contracts Polio after Shot of Serum," *Idaho State Journal,* April 26, 1955; "Polio Ends Life of School Girl," *Idaho State Journal,* April 27, 1955.

83 Idaho cases: L. J. Peterson, W. W. Benson, and F. O. Graeber, Vaccination-induced poliomyelitis in Idaho: Preliminary report of experience with Salk poliomyelitis vaccine, *Journal of the American Medical Association* 159 (1955): 241–44; "U.S. Health Experts Arrive Here to Probe City's Two Polio Cases," *Idaho State Journal,* April 28, 1955; "Official Hints Vaccine Role in Polio Out-

break; Study Begins of Cases," *Idaho Falls Post-Register*, May 1, 1955; "2nd Vaccinated Idaho Child Dies of Polio: Guard Flies Iron Lung," *Idaho Falls Post-Register*, May 2, 1955; "Idaho Officials Halt Shots 'Til Safety Assured," *Idaho Falls Post-Register*, May 3, 1955; "Polio Cases Due Visit of Officers," *Idaho Falls Post-Register*, May 3, 1955; "Vaccine Batch Appears Cause of Idaho Polio," *Idaho Falls Post-Register*, May 5, 1955: "Vaccine Fault Indicated in Idaho's Polio," *Idaho Falls Post-Register*, May 5, 1955; "Release Halted for Short Time," *Idaho Falls Post-Register*, May 7, 1955; "Two More Polio Cases Develop," *Idaho Falls Post-Register*, May 7, 1955; "Idaho Polio Toll Hits 12," *Idaho Falls Post-Register*, May 8, 1955; "Polio Strikes Driggs Girl," *Idaho Falls Post-Register*, May 9, 1955; "Danny Eggers Succumbs to Polio after Shot," *Idaho Falls Post-Register*, May 11, 1955.

84 Description of Alexander Langmuir: Interview with Neal Nathanson, August 28, 1998.

84 Distribution of Cutter's vaccine: N. Nathanson and A. D. Langmuir, The Cutter Incident: Poliomyelitis following formaldehyde-inactivated poliovirus vaccination in the United States during the spring of 1955, II: Relationship of poliomyelitis to Cutter vaccine, *American Journal of Hygiene* 78 (1963): 29–60.

85 Langmuir and the Epidemic Intelligence Service: Langmuir cited in A. D. Langmuir and J. M. Andrews, Biological warfare defense, 2: The Epidemiologic Intelligence Service of the Communicable Diseases Center, *American Journal of Public Health* 42 (1952): 235–38; A. R. Hinman and S. B. Thacker, Invited commentary on "The Cutter Incident": Poliomyelitis following formaldehyde-inactivated poliovirus vaccination in the United States during the spring of 1955, II: Relationship of poliomyelitis to Cutter vaccine, *American Journal of Epidemiology* 142 (1995): 107–8.

87 Manley Shaw: M. B. Shaw, K. Sunada, and I. A. Hopkey, Clinical study of four hundred twenty-five Idaho vaccine recipients in 1955, *American Journal of Diseases and Childhood* 96 (1958): 58–63.

87 Langmuir reaction to Atlanta cases: A. D. Langmuir, The surveillance of communicable diseases of national importance, *New England Journal of Medicine* 268 (1963): 182–92.

89 Robert Cutter on vaccine: Cited in Spencer Klaw, "Salk Vaccine: The Business Gamble," *Fortune*, September 1955, 177.

89 Habel-Tripp investigation: All facts about the investigation of Cutter Laboratories by Karl Habel and William Tripp and all quotes by Karl Habel were obtained from the following three sources: K. Habel and W. Tripp, Inspection of Cutter Laboratories, April 28–May 12, 1955, sent to William Workman, Laboratory of Biologics Control (provided by Dr. Martha Lepow); interim reports by Habel and Tripp filed May 1 and 3, 1955 (provided by Dr. Martha Lepow); reporter's transcript, *Gottsdanker v. Cutter Laboratories*, District Court of Appeal of the State of California, First Appellate District, 1 Civ. 18,413 and 18,414.

90 Habel and Tripp description and backgrounds: Interviews with Ruth Kirchstein, October 7, 1998, and April 20, 1999; reporter's transcript, *Gottsdanker v. Cutter Laboratories,* District Court of Appeal of the State of California, First Appellate District, 1 Civ. 18,413 and 18,414.

93 "A lot of tragedy": Interview with Ruth Kirchstein, October 7, 1998.

94 Meeting at the National Institutes of Health, April 29 and 30: All quotes from this two-day meeting were obtained from a complete transcript of the proceedings in the Library of the National Institutes of Health: Transcript of proceedings, National Institutes of Health meeting, Ad Hoc Committee on Poliomyelitis Vaccine, Bethesda, Maryland, April 29 and 30, 1955 (Washington, D.C.: Federal Reporting Company). Emphases added.

98 Letter from Enders to Sebrell, May 2, 1955: Thomas Rivers Archive, American Philosophical Society, Philadelphia, PA.

98 Vaccine postponed: B. Furman: "US Halts Flow of Polio Vaccine Pending a Study," *New York Times,* May 7, 1955, and "Polio Shot Delay Is Asked by US: May Last a Month," *New York Times,* May 8, 1955; P. Kihss, "Further Polio Shot Delay Urged Pending New Check: US Still Supports Vaccine," *New York Times,* May 9, 1955; "Recheck of Vaccines at Plants on Today," *New York Times,* May 11, 1955; "Halt!" *Time,* May 16, 1955; "Vaccine Evidence," *Time,* May 23, 1955; "Vaccine Snafu," *Time,* May 30, 1955; Fred A. Cutter, "Vaccine Crisis," *Time,* May 30, 1955; M. Gayn, Polio: Canada's way, *The Nation* 180 (1955): 476–78.

98 Suspension of vaccine in other countries: Rutty, " 'Do Something,' " 361.

98 Scheele on television: Cited in Carter, *Breakthrough,* 324–26.

99 O'Connor on Scheele: Ibid., 326.

99 Scheele on O'Connor: Ibid.

99 Release of vaccine: Leonard A. Scheele, *Public Health Service Technical Report on Salk Poliomyelitis Vaccine* (U.S. Department of Health, Education, and Welfare, June 1955); provided by Dr. Thomas Weller. Cited below as Scheele, *Technical Report.*

100 Percent of lots that contained live virus: Ibid.

100 Scheele, May 9: "Further Polio Shot Delay Urged Pending New Check: US Still Supports Vaccine," *New York Times,* May 9, 1955.

100 Habel on Cutter vaccine: K. Habel and W. Tripp, Inspection of Cutter Laboratories, April 28–May 12, 1955, sent to William Workman, Laboratory of Biologics Control; interim reports by Habel and Tripp filed May 1 and 3, 1955 (all provided by Dr. Martha Lepow).

101 Erlichman letter: I. Fulton Erlichman to James A. Shannon, December 20, 1955; National Archives and Records Administration, Southeast Regional Branch, Atlanta, GA.

101 Nathanson and PSU findings: A. Langmuir, N. Nathanson, and W. J. Hall, The

Wyeth problem: An epidemiological analysis of the occurrence of poliomyelitis in association with certain lots of Wyeth vaccine. Prepared by the Poliomyelitis Surveillance Unit, Epidemiology Branch, Communicable Diseases Center, Department of Health, Education, and Welfare, August 31, 1955.

102 Wyeth problem: Ibid. Also W. J. Hall and N. Nathanson, The Wyeth report: An epidemiologic investigation of the occurrence of poliomyelitis in association with certain lots of Wyeth vaccine, March 1957. Both the Wyeth problem and the Wyeth report were obtained from the National Archives and Records Administration, Southeast Regional Branch, Atlanta, GA; Scheele, *Technical Report;* Weller, *Growing Pathogens,* 88.

102 Nathanson conclusion: A. Langmuir, N. Nathanson, and W. J. Hall, The Wyeth problem: An epidemiological analysis of the occurrence of poliomyelitis in association with certain lots of Wyeth vaccine, August 31, 1955.

104 Nathanson on Wyeth vaccine: Interviews with Neal Nathanson, August 28, 1998, and August 18, 2003.

104 David Cutter on the Cutter Incident: Interviews with David L. Cutter, August 20, 1998, and February 11, 1999.

Chapter 6: What Went Wrong at Cutter Laboratories

The chapter centers on a congressional hearing chaired by Tennessee democrat Percy Priest: *Poliomyelitis Vaccine: Hearings before the Committee on Interstate and Foreign Commerce, House of Representatives, Eighty-Fourth Congress, First Session on Scientific Panel Presentation on Poliomyelitis Vaccine, June 22 and 23, 1955* (Washington, D.C.: United States Government Printing Office, 1955). All quotes from the Priest hearing can be found in this reference (emphases added).

105 Federal requirements regarding type 1 polio virus: Minimum Requirements: Poliomyelitis Vaccine, May 20, 1954; September 13, 1954; December 14, 1954; and April 12, 1955 (1st revision). Emphasis added.

106 Bazeley: Carter, *Breakthrough,* 141.

106 Salk regarding sediment in filtered vaccine: Letter from Jonas Salk to James A. Shannon, October 5, 1955. Thomas Rivers Archive, American Philosophical Society, Philadelphia, PA.

108 Bodian on filters: D. Bodian, Control of the manufacture of poliomyelitis vaccine, in *Poliomyelitis: Papers and discussions presented at the Fourth International Conference* (Philadelphia: J. B. Lippincott, 1958), 78–81.

108 A. J. Beale: Interview, April 19, 2001; A. J. Beale, The development of IPV, in *Vaccinia, Vaccination and Vaccinology: Jenner, Pasteur and Their Successors,* ed. S. Plotkin and B. Fantini (Paris: Elsevier, 1996), 221–27.

108 Change in government requirements for filtration: Minimum Requirements: Poliomyelitis Vaccine, November 11, 1955.

109 Change in government requirements for cell culture testing: Minimum Requirements: Poliomyelitis Vaccine, May 26, 1955.

109 Detection of live virus in Cutter's vaccine: C. Eklund, J. Bell, and R. K. Gerloff, Poliomyelitis in Idaho after use of live virus vaccine, *Public Health Reports* 73 (1958): 637–47; C. M. Eklund, W. J. Hadlow, E. G. Pickens, and R. K. Gerloff, Detecting poliovirus in vaccine lots used in Idaho in 1955, *Public Health Reports* 74 (1959): 60–66; L. P. Gebhardt and J. G. Bachtold, Isolation of virus from a commercial lot of poliomyelitis vaccine, *American Journal of Hygiene* 64 (1956): 70–73; A. D. Langmuir, N. Nathanson, and W. J. Hall, Surveillance of poliomyelitis in the United States in 1955, *American Journal of Public Health* 46 (1956): 75–88; W. B. Beardmore, A. E. Hook, W. Sarber, I. W. McLean, and A. R. Taylor, Poliomyelitis vaccine safety testing by the tissue culture method, *Journal of Immunology* 79 (1957): 489–96; J. Cornfield, M. Halperin, and F. Moore, Some statistical aspects of safety testing the Salk poliomyelitis vaccine, *Public Health Reports* 71 (1956): 1045–56.

110 Change in government requirements for monkey inoculations: Minimum Requirements: Poliomyelitis Vaccine, September 10, 1955.

110 Donald Trotter: Reporter's transcript, *Gottsdanker v. Cutter Laboratories,* District Court of Appeal of the State of California, First Appellate District, 1 Civ. 18,413 and 18,414.

110 Filtered virus in refrigerator: Interviews with Neal Nathanson, August 28, 1998, and August 18, 2003.

110 Change in minimum requirements for storage: Minimum Requirements: Poliomyelitis Vaccine, November 11, 1955. Emphasis added.

111 Salk recommends four samples: J. E. Salk, U. Krech, J. S. Youngner, B. L. Bennett, L. J. Lewis, and P. L. Bazeley, Formaldehyde treatment and safety testing of experimental poliomyelitis vaccine, *American Journal of Public Health* 44 (1954): 563–70; Salk protocol: Specifications and minimal requirements for poliomyelitis vaccine aqueous (polyvalent) as developed by Dr. Jonas E. Salk, Virus Research Laboratory, University of Pittsburgh, Pittsburgh, Pennsylvania (To be used for field studies to be conducted during 1954 under the auspices of the National Foundation for Infantile Paralysis), February 1, 1954 (provided by Dr. Martha Lepow).

112 Company inactivation data: Jonas Salk Archive, Mandeville Collection, La Jolla, California; interview with Robert Hull (responsible in 1955 for polio vaccine manufacture at Eli Lilly), August 7, 2000.

112 Ward as expert: Interview with E. A. Cutter, former lawyer for Cutter Laboratories (1968–1983) and the son of Ted Cutter, February 26, 2004.

113 Letters from Walter Ward to Jonas Salk: Jonas Salk Archive, Mandeville Collection, La Jolla, California.

113 Shannon and Scheele on errors: Steven M. Spencer, "Where Are We Now on Polio?" *Saturday Evening Post,* September 10, 1955.

113 Ward in court, 1976: *Mayer v. Cutter Laboratories*, February 24, 1976; available in Jonas Salk Archive, Mandeville Collection, La Jolla, California.

114 Senior virologist regarding Cutter's competence: Interview with Maurice Hilleman, January 19, 1998.

114 Deromedi on assigning blame: Interview with Frank Deromedi, February 11, 2000.

114 Routh on assigning blame: Interview with Robert Routh, February 11, 2000.

114 Robert Cutter on what happened at Cutter Laboratories: Cited in Morris, *Cutter Laboratories*, vol. 1, 230.

115 Winegarden on what happened at Cutter Laboratories: Cited in ibid., vol. 2, 115.

116 Lippmann: Walter Lippmann, "Polio Vaccine and Public Policy," *Washington Post*, May 10, 1955.

116 Editorial from *New England Journal of Medicine:* Narrow is the way, *New England Journal of Medicine* 252 (1955): 1096–97.

118 Firings in wake of Cutter Incident: Interviews with Ruth Kirchstein, October 7, 1998, and April 20, 1999; W. M. Blair, "Eisenhower Hails Mrs. Hobby's Job; Says She May Quit," *New York Times*, May 19, 1955; " 'Fumbling' on Polio Laid to Mrs. Hobby," *New York Times*, June 27, 1955; W. H. Lawrence, "Mrs. Hobby Quits as Welfare Head; Folsom Is Named," *New York Times*, July 14, 1955; B. Furman, "President Names Surgeon General," *New York Times*, August 3, 1956.

119 Enders and quack medicine: Cited in Carter, *Breakthrough*, 323.

119 Salk and suicide: Ibid.

120 Bodian on inactivation: D. Bodian, Control of the manufacture of poliomyelitis vaccine, in *Poliomyelitis: Papers and discussions presented at the Fourth International Conference* (Philadelphia: J. B. Lippincott, 1958), 78.

120 Parents' fears of vaccine: "Recheck of Vaccines at Plants on Today," *New York Times*, May 11, 1955; W. M. Blair: "Capital Expects a Further Delay in Polio Program," *New York Times*, May 13, 1955, and "3 Scientists Urge Inoculation Halt," *New York Times*, June 23, 1955; R. Porter, "Vaccine Lacking, City Delays Anew," *New York Times*, May 14, 1955.

120 "The nation is now badly scared": Cited in Carter, *Breakthrough*, 327; D. D. Rutstein, "How Good Is Polio Vaccine?" *Atlantic Monthly* 199 (1957): 48–51; L. J. Peterson, "Is Polio Vaccine Safe Now?" *U.S. News and World Report*, July 1, 1955.

120 American Academy of Pediatrics statement: Thomas Rivers Archive, American Philosophical Society, Philadelphia, PA. Emphasis added.

120 Scheele to Hobby: Scheele, *Technical Report*, ii.

121 Benjamin Franklin and smallpox: Cited in M. Radetsky, Smallpox: A history of its rise and fall, *Pediatric Infectious Disease Journal* 18 (1999): 85–93.

121 Lady Montagu: Cited in ibid.

122 Pasteur and rabies vaccine: S. A. Plotkin, C. E. Rupprecht, and H. Koprowski, Rabies vaccine, in Plotkin and Orenstein, *Vaccines*, 1025–26.

122 Yellow fever vaccine and hepatitis: J. P. Fox, C. Manso, H. A. Penna, and M. Para, Observations on the occurrence of icterus in Brazil following vaccination against yellow fever, *American Journal of Hygiene* 36 (1942): 68–116; M. V. Hargett and H. W. Burruss, Aqueous-base yellow fever vaccine, *Public Health Reports* 58 (1943): 505–12; W. A. Sawyer, K. F. Meyer, M. D. Eaton et al., Jaundice in army personnel in the western region of the United States and its relation to vaccination against yellow fever, *American Journal of Hygiene* 40 (1944): 35–107; L. B. Seeff, G. W. Beebe, J. H. Hoofnagle et al., A serologic follow-up of the 1942 epidemic of post-vaccination hepatitis in the United States Army, *New England Journal of Medicine* 316 (1987): 965–70.

123 Vaccine disaster in Germany: Plotkin and Orenstein, *Vaccines*, 187; F. Luelmo, BCG vaccination, *American Review of Respiratory Diseases* 125 (1982) (supplement): 70–72.

124 Polio in Boston: F. R. Philbrook and T. H. Ingalls, Poliomyelitis vaccination in Southeast Massachusetts in 1955: Influence of a single-dose of Salk vaccine, *New England Journal of Medicine* 255 (1956): 385–87; A. S. Pope, R. F. Feemster, D. E. Rosengard, F. R. B. Hopkins, B. Vanadzin, and E. W. Pattison, Evaluation of poliomyelitis vaccination in Massachusetts, *New England Journal of Medicine* 254 (1956): 110–17.

124 Polio in Chicago: H. N. Bundesen, H. M. Graning, E. L. Goldberg, and F. C. Bauer, Preliminary report and observations on the 1956 poliomyelitis outbreak in Chicago, *Journal of the American Medical Association* 163 (1957): 1604–19.

125 Polio vaccine between 1955 and 1961: N. Nathanson and J. R. Martin, The epidemiology of poliomyelitis: Enigmas surrounding its appearance, epidemiology and disappearance, *American Journal of Epidemiology* 110 (1979): 672–92; N. Nathanson, Eradication of poliomyelitis in the United States, *Reviews of Infectious Diseases* 4 (1982): 940–45; D. Salk, Eradication of poliomyelitis in the United States, II: Experience with killed poliovirus vaccine, *Reviews of Infectious Diseases* 2 (1980): 243–57; A. D. Langmuir, N. Nathanson, and W. J. Hall, Surveillance of poliomyelitis in the United States in 1955, *American Journal of Public Health* 46 (1956): 75–88; E. A. Timm, I. W. McLean Jr., C. H. Kupsky, and A. E. Hook, The nature of the formalin inactivation of poliomyelitis virus, *Journal of Immunology* 77 (1956): 444–52; A. L. Van Wezel, Present state and developments in the production of inactivated poliomyelitis vaccine, *Development of Biological Standards* 47 (1981): 7–13; A. L. Van Wezel, G. van Steenis, C. A. Hannik, and H. Cohen, New approach to the production of concentrated and purified inactivated polio and rabies tissue culture vaccines, *Development of Biological Standards* 41 (1978): 159–68; A. L. Van Wezel, G. van Steenis, P. van der Marel, and D. M. E. Osterhaus, Inactivated poliovirus vaccine: Current production methods and new developments, *Reviews of Infectious Diseases* 6

(1984): S335–S340; Center for Disease Control, Poliomyelitis Surveillance Summary 1976–1977, issued October 1977; Carter, *Breakthrough*, 354.

125 Sabin background and personality: Smith, *Patenting the Sun*, 146–48; Interviews with Hilary Koprowski, June 25, 1998, and July 28, 1998.

125 Sabin vaccine and testing: Carter, *Breakthrough*, 358–63.

126 George Dick's studies: D. S. Dane, G. W. A. Dick, J. H. Connolly, O. D. Fisher, F. McKeown, M. Briggs, R. Nelson, and D. Wilson, Vaccination against poliomyelitis with live virus vaccines, 1: A trial of TN type II vaccine, *British Medical Journal* 1 (1957): 59–74; Carter, *Breakthrough*, 358. Emphasis added.

126 Sabin vaccine vs. Salk vaccine: S. A. Plotkin, The choice between killed- and live-virus poliomyelitis immunization, *Clinical Pediatrics* 2 (1963): 289–95, and Inactivated polio vaccine for the United States: A missed vaccination opportunity, *Pediatric Infectious Disease Journal* 14 (1995): 835–39; J. L. Melnick, Advantages and disadvantages of killed and live poliomyelitis vaccines, *Bulletin of the World Health Organization* 56 (1978): 21–38; P. L. Ogra, and H. S. Faden, Poliovirus vaccines: Live or dead, *Journal of Pediatrics* 108 (1986): 1031–33.

126 Advisory committee statement regarding Sabin's vaccine: Cited in Carter, *Breakthrough*, 366–67.

126 Sabin vaccine causes paralysis: Oral poliomyelitis vaccines: Report of special advisory committee on oral poliomyelitis vaccines to the Surgeon General of the Public Health Service, *Journal of the American Medical Association* 190 (1964): 49–51; D. A. Henderson, J. J. Witte, L. Morris, and A. D. Langmuir, Paralytic disease associated with oral polio vaccines, *Journal of the American Medical Association* 190 (1964): 153–60.

127 Albert Sabin regarding his vaccine as a cause of paralysis: A. B. Sabin, Commentary on report of oral poliomyelitis vaccines, *Journal of the American Medical Association* 190 (1964): 52–55.

127 Why Sabin vaccine causes paralysis: O. M. Kew and B. K. Nottay, Molecular epidemiology of polioviruses, *Review of Infectious Diseases* 6 (1984): S499–S504; N. Kitamura, B. L. Semler, P. G. Rothberg, G. R. Larsen, C. J. Adler et al., Primary structure, gene organization and polypeptide expression of poliovirus RNA, *Nature* (London) 291 (1983): 547–53; N. La Monica, C. Meriam, and V. R. Racaniello, Mapping sequences required for mouse neurovirulence of poliovirus type 2 Lansing, *Journal of Virology* 57 (1986): 515–25; B. M. Nkowane, S. J. M. Wassilak, W. A. Orenstein, K. J. Bart, L. B. Schonberger, A. R. Hinman, and O. M. Kew, Vaccine-associated paralytic poliomyelitis: United States: 1973 through 1984, *Journal of the American Medical Association* 257 (1987): 1335–40; V. R. Racaniello and D. Baltimore, Molecular cloning of poliovirus cDNA and determination of the complete nucleotide sequence of the viral genome, *Proceedings of the National Academy of Sciences USA* 78 (1981): 4887–91; G. V. Rezapkin, W. Alexander, E. Dragunsky, M. Parker, K. Pomeroy et al., Genetic stability of Sabin type 1 strain of poliovirus: Implications for quality

control of oral poliovirus vaccine, *Virology* 245 (1998): 183–87; G. Stanway, A. J. Cann, R. Hauptmann, P. J. Hughes, R. C. Mountford, P. D. Minor, G. C. Schild, and J. W. Almond, The nucleotide sequence of poliovirus type 3 Leon alb: Comparison with poliovirus type 1, *Nucleic Acids Research* 11 (1983): 5629–43; G. Stanway, P. J. Hughes, R. C. Mountford, P. Reeve, P. D. Minor, G. C. Schild, and J. W. Almond, Comparison of the complete nucleotide sequences of the genomes of the neurovirulent poliovirus P3/Leon/37 and its attenuated vaccine derivative P3/Leon 2alb, *Proceedings of the National Academy of Sciences USA* 81 (1984): 1539–43; P. M. Strebel, R. Sutter, S. L. Cochi, R. J. Biellik, E. W. Brink et al., Epidemiology of poliomyelitis in the United States one decade after the last reported case of indigenous wild virus-associated disease, *Clinical Infectious Diseases* 14 (1992): 568–79; H. Toyoda, M. Kohara, Y. Kataoka, T. Suganuma, T. Omata, N. Imura, and A. Nomoto, Complete nucleotide sequences of all three poliovirus serotype genomes: Implication for genetic relationship, gene function and antigenic determinants, *Journal of Molecular Biology* 174 (1984): 561–85.

127 Salk letter to Langmuir: March 3, 1976; Thomas Rivers Archive, American Philosophical Society, Philadelphia, PA.

127 Polio recommendation in 1998: Recommendations of the Advisory Committee on Immunization Practices: Revised recommendations for routine poliomyelitis vaccination, *Morbidity and Mortality Weekly Report* 48 (1999): 590.

127 1958 survey: Williams, *Virus Hunters,* 271.

128 Sabin on Salk in 1948: Cited in Carter, *Breakthrough,* 91.

128 Sabin on Salk in 1953: Cited in Smith, *Patenting the Sun,* 193, 200.

128 Sabin on Salk in 1954: Cited in Carter, *Breakthrough,* 219.

129 Sabin on Salk vaccine after Winchell accusations: Ibid.

129 Sabin in response to Kempe letter: Cited in Smith, *Patenting the Sun,* 243.

129 Salk on Sabin's response to radio text: Cited in Carter, *Breakthrough,* 156.

129 Nixon and Sabin: Cited in Smith, *Patenting the Sun,* 386.

129 Sabin at the age of eighty-four: Cited in G. Johnson, "Once Again a Man with a Mission," *New York Times,* November 25, 1990.

129 Polio scientists elected to the National Academy of Sciences: Carter, *Breakthrough,* 299.

130 Thomas Rivers on Salk: Cited in ibid.

130 Thomas Weller on Salk: Interview with Thomas Weller, October 27, 1998.

130 Renato Dulbecco's Salk obituary: R. Dulbecco, Jonas Salk, *Nature* 376 (1995): 216.

Chapter 7: Cutter in Court

Unless otherwise stated, all quotes in this chapter were obtained from the reporter's transcript, *Gottsdanker v. Cutter Laboratories,* District Court of Appeal of the State of California, First Appellate District, 1 Civ. 18,413 and 18,414, November 20, 1957–January 31, 1958. Emphases added.

132 Belli and media circus: Interview with Richard Gerry, formerly of the law firm of Belli, Ashe, and Gerry, February 10, 1999.

132 Belli cartoon: *San Diego Union Tribune*, July 9, 1996.

132 King of Torts: Belli, *Life*, 153.

132 Belli clients: Belli, *Life*.

133 Belli obituary: *San Francisco Chronicle*, July 19, 1996.

133 Gerry on Belli: Interview with Richard Gerry, February 10, 1999.

133 Belli on suing Cutter: Belli, *Life*, 209.

133 Lawsuits against other manufacturers: Interviews with James Gault and Scott Conley, February 11, 1999, and Richard Gerry, February 10, 1999.

135 Anne Gottsdanker on walking in front of the jury: Interview with Anne Gottsdanker, June 12, 2000.

137 Ward remembered: Interview with James Gault and Scott Conley, February 11, 1999.

139 Belli on cover-up: Belli, *Life*, 211.

140 Description of Sedgwick: Interview with James Gault and Scott Conley, February 11, 1999.

142 Description of Sedgwick: Ibid.

143 Gault on Sedgwick: Interview with James Gault, February 11, 1999.

144 Belli on Stanley: Belli, *Life*, 216.

145 Conley on countersuit: Interview with Scott Conley, February 11, 1999.

146 Venezuelan equine encephalitis vaccine: D. G. Smith, H. K. Mamay, R. G. Marshall, and J. C. Wagner. Venezuelan equine encephalomyelitis: Laboratory aspects of fourteen human cases following vaccination and attempts to isolate the virus from the vaccine, *American Journal of Hygiene* 63 (1956): 150–64; L. S. Sutton and C. C. Brooke, Venezuelan equine encephalomyelitis due to vaccination in man, *Journal of the American Medical Association* 155 (1954): 1473–76.

150 Fred Cutter at trial: Memoir of Fred Cutter, January 1958 (provided by David L. Cutter).

152 Gault on verdict: Interview with James Gault, February 11, 1999.

152 Belli on verdict: Belli, *Life*, 219.

152 Letter from Belli to Salk: January 20, 1958; Jonas Salk Archive, Mandeville Collection, University of California at San Diego, La Jolla, California.

152 Letter from Salk to Belli: January 22, 1958; Jonas Salk Archive, Mandeville Collection, University of California at San Diego, La Jolla, California.

153 Letter from Robert Cutter to shareholders: February 18, 1958 (provided by David L. Cutter).

153 Reaction of jurors and judge to verdict: Michael Harris, "Cutter Verdict: Families Awarded Total of $147,300," *San Francisco Chronicle*, Saturday, January 18, 1958; "Cutter in Court," *Time*, January 27, 1958.

Chapter 8: Cigars, Parasites, and Human Toes

The development of liability law as constructed in this chapter was derived principally from Peter Huber, *Liability*. The best summary of the legal issues in the Gottsdanker verdict can be found in *Gottsdanker v. Cutter Laboratories*, 6 Cal. Rptr. 320 (Cal. Ct. App. 1960). All quotes from Wallace Sedgwick during his appeal of the Gottsdanker verdict are contained in *Gottsdanker v. Cutter Laboratories*, Opening brief of defendant and appellant Cutter Laboratories, District Court of Appeal, State of California, First Appellate District, 1 Civ. 18,413 and 18,414, and *Fitzgerald v. Cutter Laboratories*, Opening brief of defendant and appellant Cutter Laboratories, District Court of Appeal, State of California, First Appellate District, Division Two, Civil nos. 19,104, 19,105, 19,106, 19,107. All quotes from plaintiff's attorneys in response to Sedgwick's appeal are contained in *Gottsdanker v. Cutter Laboratories*, Brief for plaintiffs and respondents, supplemental brief, and amici curiae brief for appellants Gottsdanker and Phipps, District Court of Appeal, State of California, First Appellate District, 1 Civ. 18,413 and 18,414, and *Fitzgerald v. Cutter Laboratories*, Brief for plaintiffs and respondents, District Court of Appeal, State of California, First Appellate District, Division Two: Civil nos. 19,104, 19,105, 19,106, 19,107.

154 Huber on more liability: Huber, *Liability*, 221.

154 Belli on impact of Gottsdanker decision: Belli, *Life*, 218.

155 Medieval England: *Gottsdanker v. Cutter Laboratories*, Opening brief of defendant and appellant Cutter Laboratories, District Court of Appeal, State of California, First Appellate District, 1 Civ. 18,413 and 18,414.

155 Hawkins: *Hawkins v. McGee*, 84 N. H. 114.

155 Jones: *Jones v. Bright*, 5 Bing. 531.

156 Klein: *Klein v. Duchess Sandwich Co.*, 14 Cal. 2d 272.

156 Boyd: *Boyd v. Coca-Cola Bottling Works*, 177 SW 80.

157 Pillars: *Pillars v. R. J. Reynolds Tobacco Co.*, 78 S. 365.

157 Vaccarezza: Vaccarezza v. Sanguinetti, 163 P.2d 470.

157 Massengill: E. M. K. Geiling and P. R. Cannon, Pathologic effects of elixir of sulfanilamide (diethylene glycol) poisoning, *Journal of the American Medical Association* 111 (1938): 919–26; P. N. Leech, Elixir of sulfanilamide—Massengill, *Journal of the American Medical Association* 109 (1937): 1531–39; R. Steinbrook, Testing medications in children, *New England Journal of Medicine* 347 (2002): 1462–70; P. M. Wax, Elixirs, diluents, and the passage of the 1938 federal Food, Drug, and Cosmetic Act, *Annals of Internal Medicine* 122 (1995): 456–

61; "Fatal Elixir Seized as Adulterated," *New York Times,* October 30, 1937; " 'Death Drug' Hunt Covered 15 States," *New York Times,* November 26, 1937.

158 Massengill's development strategy: Cited in P. M. Wax, Elixirs, diluents, and the passage of the 1938 federal Food, Drug, and Cosmetic Act, *Annals of Internal Medicine* 122 (1995): 456–61.

158 Massengill president: Cited in Huber, *Liability,* 24.

158 Escola: *Escola v. Coca-Cola Bottling Co. of Fresno,* 150 P.2d 436. Emphasis added in quote.

161 Judge's instruction: Emphasis added.

162 Austin Smith: Cited in "The Effect on the Retail Pharmacist of the Implied Warranty Decision against Cutter," speech given by Wallace Sedgwick to pharmacists (provided by David L. Cutter).

162 Beesley: Cited in Belli, *Life,* 219.

163 American College of Physicians: *Gottsdanker v. Cutter Laboratories,* Opening brief, petition for rehearing, amicus curiae brief of American College of Physicians, amicus curiae brief of the American Pharmaceutical Association in support of defendant and appellant Cutter Laboratories, District Court of Appeal, State of California, First Appellate District, 1 Civ. 18,413 and 18,414.

165 *Yale Law Journal:* The Cutter Vaccine Incident: A case study of manufacturer's liability without fault in tort and warranty, *Yale Law Journal* 65 (1955): 262–73.

166 Cutter Laboratories after the tragedy: "How Cutter Came Back," *Business Week,* February 24, 1962; Cutter Laboratories Annual Reports, 1955–1962 (provided by David L. Cutter).

167 Brian May: Belli, *Life,* 220–21; "Young Polio Victim Receives $600,000," *Sacramento Union,* June 27, 1961.

167 Belli on May: Belli, *Life,* 222.

167 Robert Cutter letter to shareholders: Annual report from Cutter Laboratories, 1961.

168 Belli on Cutter's survival: Belli, *Life,* 222.

168 Belli on pharmaceutical industry: Ibid., 219.

168 Bendectin: The two best sources for information on Bendectin are Green, *Bendectin,* and Huber, *Junk Science,* 111–29.

169 *National Enquirer:* Cited in Green, *Bendectin,* 134.

169 Bendectin scientific studies: P. J. Aselton and H. Jick, Additional follow-up of congenital limb disorders in relation to Bendectin use, *Journal of the American Medical Association* 250 (1983): 33–34; R. L. Brent, Bendectin and intraventricular septal defects, *Teratology* 32 (1985): 317–18; W. A. Check, CDC study: No evidence for teratogenicity of Bendectin, *Journal of the American Medical Association* 242 (1979): 2518; G. Koren, A. Pastuszak, and S. Ito, Drugs in pregnancy, *New England Journal of Medicine* 338 (1998): 1128–37; P. M. McKeigue, S. H.

Lamm, S. Linn, and J. S. Kutcher, Bendectin and birth defects, I: A meta-analysis of the epidemiologic studies, *Teratology* 50 (1994): 27–37; J. Michaelis, H. Michaelis, E. Gluck, and S. Koller, Prospective study of suspected associations between certain drugs administered during early pregnancy and congenital malformations, *Teratology* 27 (1983): 57–64; A. A. Mitchell, L. Rosenberg, S. Shapiro, and D. Stone, Birth defects related to Bendectin use in pregnancy, I: Oral clefts and cardiac defects, *Journal of the American Medical Association* 245 (1981): 2311–14; A. A. Mitchell, P. J. Schwingl, L. Rosenberg et al., Birth defects in relation to Bendectin use in pregnancy, II: Pyloric stenosis, *American Journal of Obstetrics and Gynecology* 147 (1983): 737–42; S. Morelock, R. Hingsom, H. Kayne et al., Bendectin and fetal development, *American Journal of Obstetrics and Gynecology* 142 (1982): 209–13; S. Shapiro, O. P. Heinonen, V. Siskind et al., Antenatal exposure to doxylamine succinate and dicyclomine hydrochloride (Bendectin) in relation to congenital malformation, perinatal mortality rate, birth weight, and intelligence quotient score, *American Journal of Obstetrics and Gynecology* 128 (1977): 480–85; P. H. Shiono and M. A. Klebanoff, Bendectin and human congenital malformations, *Teratology* 40 (1989): 151–55; S. Zierler and K. J. Rothman, Congenital heart disease in relation to maternal use of Bendectin and other drugs in early pregnancy, *New England Journal of Medicine* 313 (1985): 347–52.

170 Ritchwald: Cited in R. L. Brent, The Bendectin saga: Another American tragedy, *Teratology* 27 (1983): 283.

170 Spokesman for Merrell Dow: Cited in Huber, *Junk Science*, 128.

170 Taj Mahal: Green, *Bendectin*, 328.

171 Breast implants: The best single source for information about breast implants and consequent litigation is Angell, *Science on Trial*.

171 Breast implants, scientific studies: C. J. Burns, T. J. Laing, B. W. Gillespie et al., The epidemiology of scleroderma among women: Assessment of risk from exposure to silicone and silica, *Journal of Rheumatology* 23 (1996): 1904–11; S. M. Edworthy, L. Martin, S. G. Barr et al., A clinical study of the relationship between silicone breast implants and connective tissue disease, *Journal of Rheumatology* 25 (1998): 254–60; S. Gabriel, W. M. O'Fallon, L. T. Kurland et al., Risk of connective-tissue diseases and other disorders after breast implantation, *New England Journal of Medicine* 330 (1994): 1697–1702; S. E. Gabriel, Breast implants and connective-tissue diseases, *New England Journal of Medicine* 331 (1994): 1233–34; J. A. Goldman, J. Greenblatt, R. Joines et al., Breast implants, rheumatoid arthritis, and connective tissue diseases in a clinical practice, *Journal of Clinical Epidemiology* 48 (1995): 571–82; C. H. Hennekens, I. M. Lee, N. R. Cook et al., Self-reported breast implants and connective-tissue diseases in female health professionals, *Journal of the American Medical Association* 275 (1996): 616–21; A. Levine, Breast implants and connective-tissue diseases, *New England Journal of Medicine* 331 (1994): 1233; J. Sanchez-

Guerrero, G. A. Colditz, E. W. Karlson et al., Silicone breast implants and the risk of connective-tissue diseases and symptoms, *New England Journal of Medicine* 332 (1995): 1666–70; B. Strom, M. M. Reidenberg, B. Freundlich, and R. Schinnar, Breast silicone implants and risk of systemic lupus erythematosus, *Journal of Clinical Epidemiology* 47 (1994): 1211–14; F. Wolfe and J. Anderson, Silicone filled breast implants and the risk of fibromyalgia and rheumatoid arthritis, *Journal of Rheumatology* 26 (1999): 2025–28; Institute of Medicine, *Safety of Silicone Breast Implants* (National Academy of Sciences Press, 1999).

172 Flowers: Cited in Andrew Skolnick, Key witness against morning sickness drug faces scientific fraud charges, *Journal of the American Medical Association* 263 (1990): 1469.

172 Incidence of dehydration doubles: Ibid., 1473.

172 Industry response regarding drugs for pregnant women: Huber, *Junk Science,* 128.

173 Wells: *Wells v. Ortho Pharmaceutical Corp.,* 788 F.2d 741 (11th Cir. 1986); J. L. Gastwirth, The need for careful evaluation of epidemiological evidence in product liability cases: A reexamination of Wells v. Ortho and Key Pharmaceuticals, *Law, Probability, and Risk* 2 (2003): 151–89.

173 Spermicidal jelly, scientific study: S. Shapiro, D. Slone, O. P. Heinonen et al. Birth defects and vaginal spermicides, *Journal of the American Medical Association* 247 (1982): 2381–84.

173 *New York Times* editorial on spermicidal jelly decision: "Federal Judges vs. Science," *New York Times,* December 27, 1986.

173 *New England Journal of Medicine* editorial: Cited in ibid.

174 Judith Haimes: "Judge Rejects Damage Award to Psychic," *Washington Post,* August 9, 1986.

175 Thalidomide: R. Brynner and T. Stephens, *Dark Remedy: The Impact of Thalidomide and Its Revival as a Vital Medicine* (New York: Perseus Publishing, 2001).

175 William McBride: W. McBride, P. H. Vardy, and J. French, Effects of scopolamine hydrobromide on the development of the chick and rabbit embryo, *Australian Journal of Biological Sciences* 35 (1982): 173–78; Andrew Skolnick, Key witness against morning sickness drug faces scientific fraud charges, *Journal of the American Medical Association* 263 (1990): 1469.

176 Alan Done: Green, *Bendectin,* 280.

176 Trauma and cancer: Huber, *Junk Science,* 40–51; G. R. Monkman, G. Orwoll, and J. C. Ivins, Trauma and oncogenesis, *Mayo Clinic Proceedings* 49 (1974): 157–63.

177 Russ Herman: Cited in Huber, *Junk Science,* 215.

177 Huber on suing the stranger: Huber, *Liability,* 189.

Chapter 9: Death for the Lambs

This chapter focuses on the National Vaccine Injury Compensation Program and its strengths and limitations. The best single source for information about this program is G. Evans, D. Harris, and E. M. Levine, Legal issues, in Plotkin and Orenstein, *Vaccines*.

178 Changes in vaccine regulation: Hilts, *Protecting America's Health;* N. Wade, Division of Biologic Standards: Scientific management questioned, *Science* 175 (1972): 966–70; Congressional Record—Senate, December 8, 1971, 45391–98; interview with William Egan, Centers for Biological Evaluation and Research, March 15, 2004.

179 "First coordinated national response": A. R. Hinman and S. B. Thacker, Invited commentary on "The Cutter Incident": Poliomyelitis following formaldehyde-inactivated poliovirus vaccination in the United States during the spring of 1955, II: Relationship of poliomyelitis to Cutter vaccine, *American Journal of Epidemiology* 142 (1995): 107–8; Etheridge, *Sentinel for Health*, 73–78.

179 Pertussis vaccine as cause of brain damage: M. Kulenkampff, J. S. Schwartzman, and J. Wilson, Neurological complications of pertussis inoculation, *Archives of Diseases of Childhood* 49 (1974): 46–49.

180 Tertussis in U.S.: Plotkin and Orenstein, *Vaccines*, 480.

180 Impact of stopping pertussis vaccine in England: E. J. Gangarosa, A. M. Galazka, C. R. Wolfe et al., Impact of anti-vaccine movements on pertussis control: The untold story, *Lancet* 351 (1998): 356–61.

180 Impact of stopping pertussis vaccine in Japan: Ibid.

181 Pertussis vaccine litigation: R. Manning, Economic impact of product liability in US prescription drug markets, *International Business Lawyer,* March 2001, 104–9, and Changing rules in tort law and the market for childhood vaccines, *Journal of Law and Economics* 37 (1994): 247–75; *Medical World News*, September 27, 1984, 15.

181 Pertussis vaccine, scientific studies: American Academy of Pediatrics, Committee on Infectious Diseases, The relationship between pertussis vaccine and brain damage: Reassessment, *Pediatrics* 88 (1991): 397–400, and The relationship between pertussis vaccine and central nervous system sequelae: Continuing assessment, *Pediatrics* 97 (1996): 279–81; J. D. Cherry, Acellular pertussis vaccines: A solution to the pertussis problem, *Journal of Infectious Diseases* 168 (1993): 21–24; J. D. Cherry and P. Olin, The science and fiction of pertussis vaccines, *Pediatrics* 104 (1999): 1381–84; Child Neurology Society, Pertussis immunization and the central nervous system, *Annals of Neurology* 29 (1991): 458–60; J. L. Gale, P. B. Thapa, S. G. F. Wassilak et al., Risk of serious acute neurological illness after immunization with diphtheria-tetanus-pertussis vaccine: A population-based case-control study, *Journal of the American Medical*

Association 271 (1994): 37–41; E. J. Gangarosa, A. M. Galazka, C. R. Wolfe et al., Impact of anti-vaccine movements on pertussis control: The untold story, *Lancet* 351 (1998): 356–61; G. S. Golden, Pertussis vaccine and injury to the brain, *Journal of Pediatrics* 116 (1990): 854–61; C. P. Howson and H. V. Fineberg, The ricochet of magic bullets: Summary of the Institute of Medicine report, Adverse Effects of Pertussis and Rubella Vaccines, *Pediatrics* 89 (1992): 318–39; S. S. Long, A. DeForest, D. G. Smith et al., Longitudinal study of adverse reactions following diphtheria-tetanus-pertussis vaccine in infancy, *Pediatrics* 85 (1990): 294–302; K. R. Wentz and E. K. Marcuse, Diphtheria-tetanus-pertussis vaccine and serious neurologic illness: An updated review of the epidemiologic evidence, *Pediatrics* 87 (1991): 287–97.

181 Decrease in number of companies making pertussis vaccine: Diphtheria-tetanus-pertussis vaccine shortage—United States, *Morbidity and Mortality Weekly Report* 33 (1984): 695–96.

181 Toner: *Toner v. Lederle Laboratories,* 779 F.2d 1429 (9th Cir. 1986); *Toner v. Lederle Laboratories,* Idaho 732 P.2d 297.

182 National Vaccine Injury Compensation Program: G. Evans, D. Harris, and E. M. Levine, Legal issues, in Plotkin and Orenstein, *Vaccines.*

183 Vaccine shortages: J. Cohen, U.S. vaccine supply falls seriously short, *Science* 295 (2002): 1998–2001; National Vaccine Advisory Committee, Strengthening the supply of routinely recommended vaccines in the United States: Recommendations of the National Vaccine Advisory Committee, *Journal of the American Medical Association* 290 (2003): 3122–28.

183 Influenza epidemic, 2003–2004: Data presented to the Advisory Committee for Immunization Practices, Centers for Disease Control and Prevention, June 23, 2004.

183 Influenza vaccine shortage in 2004: A. Pollack, "U. S. Will Miss Half Its Supply of Flu Vaccine: British Suspend License of Factory Making It," *New York Times,* October 6, 2004; M. Uhlman and S. Burling, "Flu-Shot Supplies Are Cut in Half," *Philadelphia Inquirer,* October 6, 2004.

184 CDC recommendations: National Vaccine Advisory Committee, Strengthening the supply of routinely recommended vaccines in the United States: Recommendations of the National Vaccine Advisory Committee, *Journal of the American Medical Association* 290 (2003): 3122–28.

184 Vaccine economics in relation to liability concerns: The best summary of the impact of litigation on vaccine makers is Steven Garber, *Product Liability and the Economics of Pharmaceuticals and Medical Devices* (Santa Monica, CA: RAND, 1993). Other sources include the following: G. Evans, D. Harris, and E. M. Levine, Legal issues, in Plotkin and Orenstein, *Vaccines;* Institute for Medicine, *Financing Vaccines in the 21st Century: Assuring Access and Availability* (Washington, D.C.: National Academies Press, 2003); R. Manning, Eco-

nomic impact of product liability in US prescription drug markets, *International Business Lawyer*, March 2001, 104–9, and Changing rules in tort law and the market for childhood vaccines, *Journal of Law and Economics* 37 (1994): 247–75; J. M. Wood, "Litigation Could Make Vaccines Extinct," *The Scientist*, January 19, 2004; R. P. Wenzel, The antibiotic pipeline: Challenges, costs, and values, *New England Journal of Medicine* 351 (2004): 523–26.

185 Children die from vaccines inadvertently contaminated with bacteria: G. S. Wilson, *The Hazards of Immunization* (New York: Althone Press, 1967), 75–84.

185 Thimerosal, scientific studies: N. Andrews, E. Miller, A. Grant, J. Stowe, V. Osborne, and B. Taylor, Thimerosal exposure in infants and developmental disorders: A retrospective cohort study in the United Kingdom does not show a causal association, *Pediatrics* 114 (2004): 584–91; W. J. Barbaresi, S. K. Katusic, R. C. Colligan, A. L. Weaver, and S. J. Jacobsen, The incidence of autism in Olmsted County, Minnesota, 1976–1997, *Archives of Pediatrics and Adolescent Medicine* 159 (2005): 37–44; J. Heron, J. Golding, and ALSPAC Study Team, Thimerosal exposure in infants and developmental disorders: A prospective cohort study in the United Kingdom does not show a causal association, *Pediatrics* 114 (2004): 577–83; A. Hviid, M. Stellfeld, J. Wohlfahrt, and M. Melbye, Association between thimerosal-containing vaccine and autism, *Journal of the American Medical Association* 290 (2003): 1763–66; Institute of Medicine, *Thimerosal and Autism* (Washington, D.C.: National Academies Press, 2004); S. Parker, B. Schwartz, J. Todd, and L. K. Pickering, Thimerosal-containing vaccines and autistic spectrum disorder: A critical review of published original data, *Pediatrics* 114 (2004): 793–804; T. Verstraeten, R. L. Davis, F. DeStefano et al., Safety of thimerosal-containing vaccines: A two-phased study of computerized health maintenance organization databases, *Pediatrics* 112 (2003): 1039–48.

186 Lyme vaccine: Centers for Disease Control and Prevention, Recommendations for the use of Lyme disease vaccine, *Morbidity and Mortality Weekly Report* 48 (1999): RR-7; S. L. Lathrop, R. Ball, P. Haber et al., Adverse event reports following vaccination for Lyme disease: December 1998–July 2000, *Vaccine* 20 (2002): 1603–8; L. H. Sigal, J. M. Zahradnik, P. Lavin et al., A vaccine consisting of recombinant Borrelia burgdorferi outer surface protein A to prevent Lyme disease, *New England Journal of Medicine* 339 (1998): 216–22; A. C. Steere, V. K. Sikand, F. Meurice et al., Vaccination against Lyme disease with recombinant Borrelia burgdorferi outer-surface lipoprotein A with adjuvant, *New England Journal of Medicine* 339 (1998): 209–15.

188 GBS: http://www.cdc.gov/groupbstrep.

188 GBS vaccine: C. J. Baker, M. A. Rench, M. S. Edwards et al., Immunization of pregnant women with a polysaccharide vaccine of group B streptococcus, *New England Journal of Medicine* 319 (1988): 1180–85.

188 Pharmaceutical company executive on GBS vaccine: Interview with Alan Shaw, formerly in the Division of Virus and Cell Biology, Merck Research Laboratories, January 16, 2004.

189 GBS-infected boy: Offit, personal communication with colleagues.

189 Pharmaceutical company executive on vaccine profits: Interview with Emilio Emini, former director of vaccine research and development, Merck Research Laboratories, January 16, 2004.

189 Vaccine revenues: Interview with Kevin Connelly, Merck Vaccine Division, February 2003.

Epilogue

193 Interview with Anne Gottsdanker, June 12, 2000.

Selected Bibliography

Angell, Marsha. *Science on Trial: The Clash of Medical Evidence and the Law in the Breast Implant Case.* New York: W. W. Norton, 1996.

Belli, Melvin. *The Belli Files: Reflections on the Wayward Law.* Englewood Cliffs, NJ: Prentice-Hall, 1983.

——. *Belli for Your Malpractice Defense.* Oradell, NJ: Medical Economics, 1986.

——. *Melvin Belli: My Life on Trial.* New York: William Morrow, 1976.

Benison, Saul. *Tom Rivers: Reflections on a Life in Medicine and Science.* Cambridge: MIT Press, 1967.

Berg, Roland. *Polio and Its Problems.* Philadelphia: J. B. Lippincott, 1948.

Black, Kathryn. *In the Shadow of Polio.* Reading, MA: Addison-Wesley, 1996.

Carter, Richard. *Breakthrough: The Saga of Jonas Salk.* New York: Trident Press, 1966.

——. *The Gentle Legions: National Voluntary Health Organizations in America.* New Brunswick, NJ: Transactions Publishers, 1992.

Daniel, Thomas M., and Frederick C. Robbins, eds. *Polio.* Rochester, NY: University of Rochester Press, 1997.

Davis, Fred. *Passage through Crisis: Polio Victims and Their Families.* New Brunswick, NJ: Transactions Publishers, 1991.

De Kruif, Paul. *Microbe Hunters.* New York: Harcourt, Brace, 1926.

——. *The Sweeping Wind.* New York: Harcourt, Brace, and World, 1962.

Emerson, Haven. *A Monograph on the Epidemic of Poliomyelitis (Infantile Paralysis).* New York: Arno Press, 1977.

Etheridge, Elizabeth. *Sentinel for Health: A History of the Centers for Disease Control.* Berkeley: University of California Press, 1992.

Francis, Thomas. *Evaluation of the 1954 Field Trial of Poliomyelitis Vaccine: Final Report.* Ann Arbor: University of Michigan Press, 1957.

Gabler, Neal. *Winchell: Gossip, Power, and the Culture of Celebrity.* New York: Vintage Books, 1994.

Goodwin, Doris Kearns. *No Ordinary Time: Franklin and Eleanor Roosevelt: The Home Front in World War II.* New York: Touchstone, 1995.

Gould, Tony. *A Summer Plague: Polio and Its Survivors.* New Haven and London: Yale University Press.

Green, Michael D. *Bendectin and Birth Defects: The Challenges of Mass Toxic Substances Litigation.* Philadelphia: University of Pennsylvania Press, 1996.

Hargrove, Jim. *The Story of Jonas Salk and the Discovery of the Polio Vaccine.* Chicago: Children's Press, 1990.

Hilts, Philip. *Protecting America's Health: The FDA, Business, and One Hundred Years of Regulation.* New York: Alfred A. Knopf, 2003.

Holton, Gerald, ed. *The Twentieth Century Sciences: Studies in the Biography of Ideas.* New York: W. W. Norton, 1972.

Howe, Howard A., and David Bodian, eds. *Neural Mechanisms in Poliomyelitis.* London: Oxford University Press, 1942.

Huber, Peter. *Galileo's Revenge: Junk Science in the Courtroom.* New York: Basic Books, 1991.

——. *Liability: The Legal Revolution and Its Consequences.* New York: Basic Books, 1988.

Klein, Aaron. *Trial by Fury.* New York: Charles Scribner's Sons, 1972.

Koprowski, Hilary, and Michael B. A. Oldstone, eds. *Microbe Hunters: Then and Now.* Bloomington, IL: Medi-Ed Press, 1996.

Leuchtenburg, William. *A Troubled Feast: American Society since 1945.* Boston: Little, Brown, 1973.

Marks, Harry. *The Progress of Experiment: Science and Therapeutic Reform in the United States, 1900–1990.* Cambridge: Cambridge University Press, 1997.

Morris, Gabrielle. *Cutter Laboratories, 1897–1972: A Dual Trust,* vols. 1 and 2. Berkeley: Regents of the University of California, 1975. Located in Regional Oral History Office, Bancroft Library, University of California, Berkeley.

Ohern, Elizabeth Moot. *Profiles of Pioneer Women Scientists.* Washington, D.C.: Acropolis Books, 1985.

Paul, John. *A History of Poliomyelitis.* New Haven and London: Yale University Press, 1971.

Plotkin, Stanley A., and Walter A. Orenstein, eds. *Vaccines,* 4th ed. Philadelphia: Saunders, 2004.

Radetsky, Peter. *The Invisible Invaders: The Story of the Emerging Age of Viruses.* Boston: Little, Brown, 1991.

Rogers, Naomi. *Dirt and Disease: Polio Before FDR*. New Brunswick, NJ: Rutgers University Press, 1992.

Rutty, Christopher. " 'Do Something! . . . Do Anything!' Poliomyelitis in Canada, 1927–1962." Graduate thesis, University of Toronto, 1995.

Sass, Edmund. *Polio's Legacy: An Oral History*. Lanham, MD: University Press of America, 1996.

Seavey, Nina G., Jane S. Smith, and Paul Wagner. *A Paralyzing Fear: The Triumph over Polio in America*. New York: TV Books, 1998.

Sherrow, Victoria. *Jonas Salk*. New York: Facts on File, 1993.

Shorter, Edward. *The Health Century*. New York: Doubleday, 1987.

Sills, David. *The Volunteers*. Glencoe, IL: Free Press, 1957.

Smith, Jane. *Patenting the Sun: Polio and the Salk Vaccine*. New York: William Morrow, 1990.

Tomlinson, Michael. *Jonas Salk*. Vero Beach, FL: Rourke Publications, 1993.

Tucker, Jonathan. *Scourge: The Once and Future Threat of Smallpox*. New York: Atlantic Monthly Press, 2001.

Weller, Thomas. *Growing Pathogens in Tissue Cultures: Fifty Years in Academic Tropical Medicine, Pediatrics, and Virology*. Canton, MA: Scientific History Publications, 2004.

Williams, Greer. *Virus Hunters*. New York: Alfred A. Knopf, 1960.

Wilson, John R. *Margin of Safety*. New York: Doubleday, 1963.

Acknowledgments

I wish to thank the following people for their generosity, kindness, and patience:

Beth Waters for her interviews of Cutter employees and victims of Cutter's vaccine and for her guidance, wisdom, thoughtfulness, insight, and humor.

Jean E. Thomson Black, senior editor, Yale University Press, for her unswerving belief in and support of this project.

Lisa Considine, Kaarel Kaljot, Patty Lund, Greg Payne, Maribeth Payne, and Angela Von Der Lippe for discussions that shaped the book's point of view.

A. J. Beale, Richard Carter, Robert Chanock, Tom Coleman, Scott Conley, David Cutter, Edward Cutter, Frank Deromedi, Edward Digardi, James Gault, Richard Gerry, Irv Gomphrect, Anne Gottsdanker, Maurice Hilleman, Robert Hull, Ruth Kirchstein, Hilary Koprowski, Neal Nathanson, Erling Norrby, John Ochsner, Stanley Plotkin, Frederick Robbins, Robert Routh, Darrell Salk, Donna Salk, Thomas Weller, and Julius Youngner for sharing their remembrances of polio and the Cutter tragedy.

Kevin Connolly, William Egan, Emilio Emini, Geoff Evans, Maurice Hilleman, Phil Hosbach, Barbara Howe, Dean Mason, Walter Orenstein, Peter Paradiso, Stanley Plotkin, Alan Shaw, and Thomas Vernon for their perspectives on the vaccine industry.

Loren Cooper, Geoff Evans, and Michael D. Green for their help with legal aspects of the Cutter court decision and the National Vaccine Injury Compensation Program.

Joanne Binkley (Center for Biologics Evaluation and Research, Food and Drug Administration), Linda Corey Claassen (Mandeville Special Collections Library, University of California, San Diego), Robert Cox (Thomas Rivers Archive, American Philosophical Society), Tom Love (Records Management Officer, National Immunizations Program), David Rose (March of Dimes Birth Defects Foundation), and Bruce Weniger (Vaccine Safety and Development Branch, National Immunization Program) for their guidance through archival material.

And Louis Bell, Nancy Biller, Bonnie Brier, Alan Cohen, Maurice Hilleman, Sam Katz, Elizabeth Layton, Nancy Librett, Jeff Lindy, Dean Mason, Don Mitchell, Charlotte Moser, Wendy Mosler, Neal Nathanson, Bonnie Offit, Carl Offit, Georges Peter, Stanley Plotkin, Adam Ratner, Darrell Salk, Alan Shaw, Roland Sutter, Kirsten Thistle, Bruce Weniger, and Amy Wilen for their careful reading of the manuscript and helpful suggestions and criticisms.

Index

Page numbers in **bold** indicate illustrations

tion of Cutter Incident, 85–86; Polio-
myelitis Surveillance Unit, 101–102
Epilepsy, pertussis vaccine hypothesis and,
180, 181
Erlichman, Fulton, 100–101
Erlichman, Pamela, 100
Escola, Gladys, 158–159
Ethylmercury, 184
Excedrin, 168
Expert witnesses, in product liability trials,
175–176
Express warranty, 155–156

Field trial (Salk vaccine), 53; consecutive-lot
requirement in, 118; consistency requirement in, 113; cost of, 52; fears of live virus,
48–49, 53; manufacturing protocol for, 44–
47, 60; National Foundation supervision
of, 60–61; number of participants, 52;
pharmaceutical companies involved in, 44,
45, 47–48; placebos in, 51–52; results of,
52–54, 116; size and scope of, 48; Winchell's broadcast, effect of, 49, 50, 51
Filtration: glass, 106, 107, 108–109; progressive, 130–131; with Seitz filters, 106, 108;
storage of filtered vaccine, 110
Flexner, Simon, 11, 21
Flowers, Charles, 172
Folk remedies, 8–9
Food and Drug Administration, 75, 158, 173,
178–179, 185, 187
Food, Drug, and Cosmetic Act of 1938, 158
Formaldehyde inactivation, 16, 18, 35, 106;
concentration in, 40, 92; time span for, 41,
43, 111–112; of Venezuelan equine
encephalitis, 146
Francis, Thomas, 30, 51, 52; field trial report
of, 54–56; investigation of Cutter vaccine,
68, 69
Franklin, Benjamin, 120–121, 122
French, Jill, 175–176
Fundraising for polio research, 20–21, 22–
24, 23, 54

Gabriel, Sherine, 171
Gard, Sven, 43
Gault, James, 142–143, 152
GBS vaccine, 188–189
Georgia Warm Springs Foundation, 20, 22
German measles, xi
German measles vaccine, 179
Gerry, Richard, 133
Gilbert, Jimmy, 84
Gittenberg, Sally, 16

Glass filtration, 106, 107, 108–109
GlaxoSmithKline, 108, 182, 187
Goodwin, Doris Kearns, 19
Gottsdanker, Anne, 1, 2, 3, 133, 135–136,
192–193
Gottsdanker, Josephine, 1, 3, 133
Gottsdanker, Robert, 133, 135
Gottsdanker v. Cutter Laboratories: appeal
of verdict, 159–164; attorneys in, 132–133,
140, 142–143; counts against Cutter, 133–
134; defense case, 143–147; implications of
liability without fault, 154, 162–165, 168,
179; instructions to jury, 148–149; jury
deliberations in, 149; plaintiffs' case, 134–
142; verdict in, 149–153
Graning, Harold, 65
Green, Edwin, 161, 162
Gregg, Alan, 56
Group A streptococcus, 193
Group B streptococcus (GBS) vaccine, 188–
189
Guérin, Camille, 123
Guilfoy, Robert, 7

Haas, Victor: dismissal of, 118; investigation
of Cutter vaccine, 67, 68, 69, 70, 94; on
safety of Salk vaccine, 49, 53
Habel, Karl: background of, 89–90; inves-
tigation of Cutter Incident, 67, 89, 90–93,
93, 100, 145; testimony in Gottsdanker
lawsuit, 145
Haimes, Judith, 173–174
Hammon, William McDowall, 68, 69, 70,
117, 119
Hammond, Jack, 36, 37
Hampil, Bettylee, 95, 96
Harrison, Elizabeth, 122
Haver-Glover Laboratories, 166
Hawkins, George, 155
Henry, Anna, 5–6
Hepatitis outbreak, yellow fever vaccine and,
122–123
Hepatitis research, on retarded children, 37
Herman, Russ, 177
Herpesviruses, 193
Hobby, Oveta Culp, 58, 61, 62, 63, 71, 101,
117, 118, 120, 144
Hollister-Stier, 166
Houlihan, Ralph, 63, 91, 110, 113
Huber, Peter, 154, 177
Hunter, John, 12

Immunity to second infection, 12
Immunologic memory, 130